EXERCISE

EXERCISE
The Facts

E. J. BASSEY and P. H. FENTEM

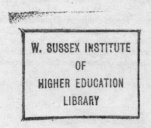

Oxford New York Toronto Melbourne
OXFORD UNIVERSITY PRESS
1981

Oxford University Press, Walton Street, Oxford OX2 6DP

London Glasgow New York Toronto
Delhi Bombay Calcutta Madras Karachi
Kuala Lumpur Singapore Hong Kong Tokyo
Nairobi Dar es Salaam Cape Town
Melbourne Wellington

and associate companies in
Beirut Berlin Ibadan Mexico City

British Library Cataloguing in Publication Data

Bassey, E J
Exercise.
1. Exercise – Physiological effect
I. Title   II. Fentem, P H
612'.76   OP301   80–41122

ISBN 0–19–286013–5 Pbk
ISBN 0–19–217716–8

Set by Filmtype Services Limited
Printed in Great Britain by
Cox & Wyman Ltd, Reading, Berks

FOREWORD

The job of the Sports Council is basically to turn Britain from a nation of Watchers into a nation of sports Doers and so I'm delighted to write a few words in praise of a book such as this one. The authors also penned the Sports Council's Research Report *The Case for Exercise*, which was published in 1978, and *Exercise for Health*, a bibliography of references collected during a literature search which proved exercise is a benefit to health.

I was glad the Sports Council took the initiative in encouraging the production of those reports, and fully back this publication. The reason why we are enthusiastic in our support is quite simple: we approve of any form of encouragement given to sports people and, more importantly, would-be sports people. Frankly, we all think sport on television is superb, but it is not enough for the human frame just to sit there and watch others in action.

As a former rugger player, I know exactly what being totally fit means. The psychological effect of knowing you can speed down the pitch without running out of steam is of enormous value to your confidence and over-all feeling of well-being. But look about you, in everyday life, and see quite young people gasping after short sprints for the bus.

Today, as an apple farmer, I still keep fit with plenty of walking. Playing golf, too, gives me tremendous pleasure and keeps the bounce in my stride. People often make cheap jokes about the hazards of exercise, and we see photographs in the newspapers of an American President who collapsed while attempting to jog. I even read an article which maintained jogging could kill. But just think of the risks we humans run by taking practically no exercise.

It's interesting this study should also be looking at obesity. Sometimes it's bad luck if people are over-fat and cannot cure the problem. More often, I imagine, they are eating the wrong foods and not burning away the surplus with honest exercise, like walking to work, or striding up the escalator – or even stretching in the morning!

Myself, I don't need the message about good health and exercise. I *know* they are allied. What I like to think comes across loud and clear is the fun that sport and recreation give to participants. No matter what your age, if you want to live a fuller life there's medical evidence to support the view that exercise pays dividends. This is why all of us at the Sports Council give this book our full support.

Dick Jeeps, C.B.E.
Chairman of the Sports Council

CONTENTS

ACKNOWLEDGEMENTS

We are indebted to the Sports Council for the financial help which made an extensive literature search possible, and to Avrille Blecher who worked with us as a research assistant during the search and collation of the literature.

We would like to thank Michael Collins and Roger Pontefract of the Sports Council (London) and Janet Mawby, the readers' adviser in the Medical School (Nottingham), for special help and encouragement. We are also grateful for the advice and information which was generously given by the following people:

Prof. Sir W. Ferguson Anderson, University of Glasgow, Glasgow; Eduardo Andrade, Confederacion Deportiva, Mexico; Prof. P.-O. Astrand, Fysiologiska institutionen, Stockholm; Dr T. E. Blecher, General Hospital, Nottingham; Dr P. Carson, City General Hospital, Stoke-on-Trent; Jean-Paul Cornic, Comité National Olympique et Sportif Français, Paris; Dr G. Cust, Health Education Council, London; Dr C. T. M. Davies, London School of Hygiene and Tropical Medicine, London; G. R. Dempster, Dept. of Environment, Housing and Community Development, Canberra; Prof. R. H. T. Edwards, University College Hospital Medical School, London; Prof. B. Ekblom, Fysiologiska institutionen, Stockholm; Ass. Prof. L.-G. Ekelund, Dept. of Clin. Physiology, Karolinska Sjukhuset, Stockholm; Prof. M. R. P. Hall, University of Southampton Faculty of Medicine, Southampton; Dr D. R. Hay, National Heart Foundation of New Zealand, Christchurch; K. J. Heather, New Zealand Council for Recreation and Sport, Wellington; Dr M. Herbert, Queen's Medical Centre, Nottingham; Prof. Dr. med. W. Hollmann, Institut für Kreislaufforschung, Cologne; Prof. J. Horak, Czechoslovak Society of Sports Medicine, Prague; Dr H. Howald, Research Institute of the Swiss School for Physical Education and Sports, Magglingen; Dr F. J. Imms, M.R.C. Environmental Physiology Unit, London; Dr T. G. Judge, South Lothian District Geriatric Service, Edinburgh; Tor Jungman, Finnish Central Sports Federation, Helsinki; Dr. J. Kane, West London Institute of Higher Education, Middlesex; Dr R. O. Keelor, President's Council on Physical Fitness and Sport, Washington; Sandy Keir, Head, Fitness Section, Recreation Canada; Ass. Prof. Asa Kilbom, National Board of Occupational Safety and Health, Stockholm; Dr K. J. Kingsbury, Amersham, Bucks; Prof. S. Kozlowski, Polish Academy of Sciences, Warsaw; Jo-Ann Lawson, Sports Federation of Canada, Ontario; Wolf Lyberg, Swedish Sports Federation, Stockholm; Prof. P. C. McIntosh, University of Otago, Dunedin, New Zealand; Keith McKerracher, President, 'Participaction' Montreal; Prof. W. Marshall, Loughborough University of Technology, Loughborough; Dr C. J. M. Martini, Queen's Medical Centre, Nottingham; Ministry of Cultural Affairs, Recreation and Social Welfare, Netherlands; Prof. J. R. A. Mitchell, General Hospital, Nottingham; V. E. S. Mkodo, National Sports Council of Tanzania, Dar es Salaam; Dr D. B. Morgan, The

General Infirmary, Leeds; Dr N. G. Norgan, University of Technology, Loughborough; Jurgen Palm, Deutscher Sportbund, Frankfurt; Ion Paun, Foreign Relations Dept., Bucharest; Dr H. Perie, Secrétariat D'État, Jeunesse et Sports, Paris; Dr M. L. Pollock, Institute for Aerobics Research, Texas; Prof. P. Puska, North Karelia County Health Administration, Kuopio, Finland; Emmanuel Rose, Danish Sports Federation, Glostrup; Mr C. Sayer, Loughborough; Prof. Schär, Institut für Sozial-und Präventivmedizin der Universität, Zurich; J. Stäuble, Swiss National Association for Physical Education, Berne; Prof. Dr. sc. med. Strauzenberg, International Federation of Sports Medicine, Kreischa, DDR: Miss A. M. Street Nielsen, Norwegian Confederation of Sports; Dr. F. Van den Bossche, Ministerie van Nationale Opvoeding en Nederlande Cultuur, Brussels; Dr J. A. White, University of Salford, Salford; Dr C. B. Wynn Parry, Royal National Orthopaedic Hospital, Middlesex; Dr A. Young, University College Hospital, London.

INTRODUCTION

Why run when you can walk?

Exercise is an ever-present part of human life. Over the centuries and across the variety of human life-styles the place of exercise and its importance for survival and well-being have varied enormously.

The wealthy have always been free to choose whether or not to exert themselves physically since their lives rested essentially on the labour of others. Until this century the less wealthy never had a choice and spent most of their day in physical work.

Now almost all of us in the affluent societies of the Western world can choose. Should we take exercise voluntarily? Alternatively we may choose not to do so; what then are the consequences of a lifetime of physical inactivity?

These questions have recently, and rather suddenly, received a great deal of attention. The spotlights of the mass media have focused upon various forms of optional exercise and the message has been lost in the blaze of publicity.

The need for exercise is preached with missionary zeal with promises of protection from killer diseases one week and scaremongering stories of deaths attributed to jogging the next. The result has been a splitting of opinions with extremists at both ends and a large number of confused people in the middle.

Athletes and Spartans have always advocated, even revered, exercise. Many more people have discovered that regular exertion can be pleasant and bring with it a sense of well-being. They want to share their discovery but coax in vain. They cannot convert those for whom physical activity is coloured by painful memories of breathlessness, aching legs, and stiffness. The attitudes which people have towards exercise are bound to be strongly influenced by their own experiences and those of others close to them. Many people still associate physical effort with poverty and an unwelcome need for labour and so despise exercise as a yoke to be cast off.

There is therefore a need for clear and honest statements to be made about what exercise does to our bodies and what its influence on health might be. The situation is not easy to explain. The links between exercise and health are not yet fully sorted out and matters have been further confused by well-meaning evangelists who in their eagerness to gain converts may distort the evidence and misrepresent the facts.

They argue by selective instance. The fact that Victor Sylvester, the ballroom-dancing celebrity, is reported in the press to have died aged 78 years of a heart attack after swimming in the sea may not have been due to the swimming. It is certainly not a sound argument to use against swimming in general even for the elderly. There are many other people in their seventies who go swimming regularly and eventually die in their beds from causes entirely unrelated to the swimming. On the other side advocates of exercise commonly say that exercise improves the efficiency of the lungs, which is an equally unsound claim. The lungs of healthy people are more than adequate for taking in oxygen and do not limit exercise capacity.

Whom should you believe? Is the emphasis on exercise just another craze, feeding on contemporary neuroses and fanatically pursued by health addicts? If so, then it will be allowed to fade into obscurity and if that happens it will be a tragedy of lost opportunities and misunderstandings.

It is to be hoped that a turning point has been reached when exercise will be better understood and recognized as a necessary cornerstone of successful living rather than a burden to be avoided. Affluence and automation have swept away the old associations between physical work and poverty for almost everyone in this country but we may now be in danger of letting high technology deprive us of the use of our legs. What of the middle-aged woman who can switch the television channels over at the touch of a button without moving from her armchair? Is there a risk that she may find that by the time she is 65 years old she can no longer get out of the armchair unassisted?

Some of the confusion in the debate has arisen because exercise is a vague word which conjures up a variety of activities whose only common element is that they require muscle power. There is exercise which is deliberately chosen for pleasure such as badminton or football, there are exercises like deep breathing and touching the toes, undertaken in the interests of better health. There is a whole range of domestic activities such as carrying shopping baskets, mowing the lawn, or walking with the dog which, whether they are pursued with vigour or reluctance, are an inescapable part of independent living for all but the very wealthy.

There is the physical effort involved in one's occupation, which is negligible for a sedentary secretary but dominates the life of a coal-face miner.

Then, whatever the original reason for taking it, exercise varies in several ways. It is possible to identify two distinct kinds of effort, continuously maintained effort and rhythmic movement. These have different effects on the body. For example, pushing the car

Fig. 1. Types of muscular activity
The physiological response to exercise depends upon the type of muscle contraction involved

Intermittent *Rhythmic*	Maintained *Isometric*
Walking	Lifting loads
Running	Carrying loads
Cycling	Supporting loads
Swimming	Pushing loads
Digging	Straining

involves continuous maintained effort whereas digging or swimming are rhythmic kinds of exercise involving intermittent effort when the muscles are rested briefly between each stroke. Both these kinds of effort can vary in both intensity and duration. Exercise must be defined in all these three ways before the arguments can begin.

Not only is there a need to define what we mean by exercise, but also to examine how attitudes towards exercise develop.

In primitive times the powerful drives of hunger or fear of physical attack put a premium on physical fitness, but in the welfare state, relieved of these pressures, man appears as a naturally lazy creature. Adults have little motivation to take exercise for its own sake and the deterioration which occurs through lack of it is so slow that it passes unnoticed. Exercise influences capacity for exercise. Do nothing and soon you will be able to do nothing else.

In addition many adults had too much exercise presented in the wrong way for the wrong reasons when they were children or adolescents and so have developed a profound antipathy to physical activity of any sort. Competitive sports allow the talented to shine but produce feelings of inferiority and inadequacy in youngsters less well endowed with the co-ordination necessary to catch or throw a ball. The product of this introduction to sport and exercise is the man or woman addicted to an armchair who fends off attempts to interest him or her in badminton or a walk in the countryside with tales of the great age of one fat indolent relative and by reference to the latest accident on the sports field.

Against this rather negative background interest in exercise has been kindled in the last few years in the hope that it might help to prevent heart disease. Claims about the 'protective' effects of exercise in heart disease have been simplified and exaggerated. They have led to large numbers of middle-aged adults jogging the streets. The jogging is good for them for many reasons provided they tackle it gradually but the motivation is a little suspect. Exercise should be a pleasant habit pursued for its own sake rather than as a dose of protective medicine.

Physical exercise should come into its own for positive rather than negative reasons. It should be fun and surely that is possible at a time when self-expression, bra-less liberation, and the pursuit of pleasure are in vogue. This has happened for some forms of exercise. But, sadly, many other forms of potentially enjoyable exercise such as cross-country running or orienteering have been tarred with the brush of puritan attitudes found in schools and so have been rejected. Yoga and keep fit classes which develop muscular control, flexibility, and strength are popular among both the young and the middle-aged. Dancing which also improves the economy of the circulation has always had a few energetic practitioners but never in the numbers who now abandon themselves to the rhythmic beat of pop music at a disco or enjoy themselves at old-time dance clubs.

The benefits of exercise have been known for a long time. The ancients knew the value of practice for developing and maintaining physical prowess of every kind. Every tribe had its games and competitions which demanded physical effort. They were played with whole-hearted enthusiasm by both children and adults alike. The immediate motive was enjoyment. The resulting muscle strength, stamina, and skill were necessary for survival, finding food, and defeating enemies, but they were also valued and prized for their own sake.

Now we have come to understand much more about the physiology of exercise, about the changes which take place in our bodies both during exercise and afterwards leading to the cumulative effects of training. Much of this was described and measured early in this century and recent research has revealed some of the changes in cell biochemistry which underlie physiological improvements in exercise capacity. Despite all this, exercise is neglected and undervalued not only by the general public but also by the medical profession. The realization that exertion this week will make the same task easier next week, which is what is meant by training, has been slow to gain wide acceptance.

The quality of life is profoundly affected by the range of physical activities which can be undertaken without strain. Our lives are limited if we do not have the physical abilities to join with others in a variety of enterprises and activities.

Your reaction may be, 'Well, I don't want to play football.' That is understandable but do you have the strength to face a country stile or a high bus platform with equanimity? Do you refuse invitations to climb to the top of a castle tower to see the view because your muscles are in such poor shape? Many people over 40 are not happy to sit on a rug on the ground or on a carpeted floor at a crowded party because they are stiff and doubt whether they have the muscle strength to get up again with dignity. The consequences of not having the physical ability to be sufficiently active to join in common enterprises are painfully obvious among the physically disabled and very old. There is no reason why the rest of us endowed with the normal array of muscles and joints should allow ourselves to drift in this direction. The deterioration in muscle strength which gives rise to the subtle disabilities described above is not an inevitable consequence of age, it is mainly due to lack of use.

A poor capacity for physical activity closes the doors on many potentially joyful pursuits, and tends to set up a vicious circle of further inactivity which leads to further deterioration and an even poorer capacity for exercise. On the other hand, if a deliberate effort is made to become more active, then things get better and better. Harder physical work can be tolerated for longer without fatigue and all daily tasks are accomplished more easily. The range of physical activities which can be safely and comfortably undertaken is extended; practical involvement in daily life is enriched; new horizons can open out; the social and psychological consequences may be far-reaching.

The exciting and comforting fact is that muscles, even after long underuse or disuse, will still increase in girth and power if exercised again. Flex them regularly for a few weeks and they will reward you, perhaps after a small initial grumble called stiffness, with a new sense of youthful well-being. The message of this book is that exercise makes good scientific sense.

It was written for a number of reasons. We believe that exercise is of undoubted value but that it is often recommended or forbidden for the wrong reasons. The publicity it receives is very confusing. Promotional material for exercise campaigns promises better health for everyone through exercise. Yet all this is tempered by tales of caution and disaster which give prominence to the risks of physical exercise for those who are not accustomed to it.

We would like to see more people taking more exercise in the informed belief that they will enjoy it and reap the benefits. We would rather they began with an understanding of what they are doing and a motivation which has more to do with a positive concern for themselves than fear of ill health. Those who plunge into jogging campaigns in ignorance and fear tend to respond erratically and give up all too soon.

During the last two or three years we have reviewed the scientific literature in a search to find the evidence that exercise is good for you. This had not been done before, so we felt uniquely placed to write a book which presented the evidence to the public. In addition we have set out the necessary background information about the response of the normal body to exercise.

The book is not about athletes who already receive almost more attention than anyone could handle. It is about and for the man and woman in the street. It explains why exercise is of benefit to almost everyone and how it can help even those who are ill, such as the bronchitic and the diabetic. It is intended for those who wish to judge for themselves whether exercise is a worthwhile human activity.

Part I

EXERCISE AND HEALTH

This section is about the immediate effects of exercise on body systems and the cumulative long-term effects of repeated exercise on normal people. It is also about the implications for positive health and well-being in various age groups and for men and women.

1

HOW THE BODY RESPONDS TO EXERCISE

Walking is exercise too

Mention of exercise brings to mind a variety of feelings which we associate with physical exertion. The pleasant feelings are hard to define, but some people find that exercise makes them feel good. For other people the overriding impression is of breathlessness and aching muscles. None of the conscious sensations tells us very much about the considerable readjustments which are taking place in the body as we move from rest to exercise.

This chapter is about the changes which take place during exercise, and how they are linked together to ensure that the increased energy is available to those parts of the muscle cell which perform the work. Fuel must be provided, waste products removed, and heat dissipated. The story is complicated in places but an understanding of what is involved is essential background for a proper appreciation of the long-term benefits of exercise.

Physical activity, especially if it is strenuous, poses a considerable challenge to the body's numerous control systems. Their purpose is to keep conditions within the body constant to within very strict limits. Human cells can only tolerate small fluctuations in temperature or acidity and need to have the concentration of substances such as oxygen, carbon dioxide, glucose, and salts kept almost constant. Nerve cells are particularly sensitive and although muscle cells are more tolerant they too have specific needs and will not function well if their surroundings depart much from the optimum.

Exercise is a challenge to the control systems because of the sudden rise in the activity of the muscle cells. The energy required by these cells can increase twenty-fold within seconds in vigorous exercise such as running. The rate of consumption of oxygen and fuel rises equally dramatically, and so does the production of heat and waste substances. All this must be accommodated smoothly without allowing fuel famines or overflow of acidic wastes to embarrass the activity of other essential tissues. Nicely co-ordinated adjustments from many body systems are needed.

If vigorous exercise such as running is to be continued for more than a few seconds the circulation and the lungs must respond. The heart must beat more rapidly and powerfully to provide the necessary increased blood flow to the dilated blood-vessels of the working muscles. Other blood-vessels in the gut and skin must constrict to compensate for the dilation in the muscles, otherwise the pressure in the whole system would drop, and flow to all parts would fail. The rate and depth of breathing must increase to ensure the flow of oxygen into the blood and to remove carbon dioxide and some of the heat. The extent of the changes which can take place in strenuous exercise is remarkable and very seldom exploited to anything like its full potential.

It is not surprising that the after-effects of prolonged vigorous exercise may last for hours and that adaptive changes may be

Fig. 2. The changes in strenuous exercise are remarkable

	Rest	Increase due to exercise
Energy release in muscle	●	●●●●●●●●●●●●●●●●●●●● (×20)
Cardiac output (total blood flow)	●	●●●●● (×5)
Muscle blood flow	●	●●●● (×4)
Ventilation	●	●●●●●●●●●● (×10)

provoked which last for days. If the exercise is undertaken repeat-edly, then the adaptive changes are cumulative; this is what happens during training, which will be described in the next chapter.

Physical work takes many forms. Exercise may be intense and over in a moment like an all-out sprint for a bus or it may be prolonged but less intense, for example a country hike which can be sustained for hours. The ways in which the body responds and the limits to energy output in these two extreme examples are quite different. In between the extremes comes exercise which is fairly vigorous but not so strenuous that it cannot be maintained for 20 or 30 minutes. Walking, running, digging, cycling, or swimming are examples. This is the kind of exercise which is most useful in training and which is most likely to bring benefits. Many people find it the most satisfying kind of exercise for this reason

and also because it feels good. The changes which it provokes will
be described under the following headings; the energy stores (fuel);
the system for exchanging oxygen for carbon dioxide in the
atmosphere (breathing); the internal transport system for these
gases and also for fuel and heat (the circulation); and the systems
for disposing of excess heat and carbon dioxide (waste disposal).

Consider an ordinary individual, not used to much exercise, who
is walking briskly, say at about 6 kilometres per hour (4 miles per
hour). This is sufficient at the least to triple the resting rate of
energy release, to produce similar increases in oxygen uptake and
ventilation of the lungs, and to raise the heart rate from 60 to 140
beats per minute. Many of us cannot maintain exercise which is
more vigorous than that for more than a few minutes.

If the walker weighs 70 kilograms (154 pounds) he will be using
up fuel and releasing energy at the rate of about 300 watts (250
kilocalories per hour). This is the rate at which three 100-watt
electric light bulbs produce energy. Since muscle cells are no more

Fig. 3. Exercise keeps us warm

The efficiency of human muscle is never greater than about 20 per cent

Combustion $\rightarrow$ Work + Heat
of fuel   20%   80%

---

efficient than most engines, only one-fifth of the energy appears as
useful work and is actually released in walking movements. Thus
energy is needed for the actual work and much more for the
obligatory release of heat. One of the good things about exercise in
a cool climate such as that of Western Europe is that it keeps you
warm.

Fuel

Movement and physical work, whether they are achieved by
man-made machines or by muscles, require a source of energy. The
energy for muscular effort or any other cell process comes from the
slow controlled breakdown of stored food, mainly glucose and fat.
The process has much in common with the combustion of petrol in a
car engine or of gas in a central-heating boiler. There is the same
release of stored energy from large organic molecules to form small
molecules, mainly carbon dioxide, the same need for oxygen from
the air. The boiler goes out without it like any fire. The difference

is that in the body the energy release is controlled by a large number of chemical substances called enzymes and so happens in a slow stepwise fashion rather than explosively. Enzymes control the rate of chemical breakdown, or synthesis, but do not themselves take part in any other way. Moreover in the body the energy is taken up and channelled through the universal energy currency of cells, adenosine triphosphate (known as ATP). The so-called high-energy phosphate bond in ATP can then split to release energy for many cell processes including the contraction of muscles.

Muscles contain enough food, stored as glycogen (polymerized glucose), to last for many minutes of running. Glycogen stores in the liver can also contribute substantial amounts of glucose. These stores are augmented and replenished by the abundant energy stored as fat in adipose tissue. Adipose tissue consists almost entirely of fat-filled cells held in a loose mesh of fibrous tissue and supplied abundantly with blood-vessels and nerves. Many people have sufficient fat to stay alive for many weeks of complete starvation; fortunately, this is seldom necessary. Adipose tissue is found packed round the abdominal organs where it gets very much in the way if surgery is necessary. It is also packed between the bundles of muscles and in layers under the skin. The 'spare tyre' is appropriately named. Women tend to keep more of it under their skin where it exaggerates their curvaceous shape. Men tend to collect it in a paunch around the abdominal organs.

The energy stores are rarely completely exhausted; there are only two circumstances worth mentioning in which this might happen. After weeks of starvation fat stores begin to run out and breakdown of protein is increasingly used as an energy supply. This is very damaging to body structures and contributes to the victim's ultimate death. The other circumstance is much less drastic and more easily reversed. At the end of a long-distance race the supply of glucose to the muscles can fail and bring the runner to a halt. There is plenty of fat left but it cannot be used unless there is a small amount of glucose present in the cells. Substances formed from glucose are needed in the complicated chain of events involved in energy release. The liver can manufacture glucose from protein but not fast enough to meet the demands of the runner.

During prolonged exercise, of even moderate intensity like a long walk or after any strenuous brief physical effort, there is a need to supplement the immediately accessible stores of fuel in the working muscle cells. This means mobilizing fat stores from depots remote from the working muscles. Several hormones are involved in this. For example, adrenalin is released during exercise and one of its effects is to release fat from adipose tissue so that it can be carried in the bloodstream to the working muscles. In the long term replenishment must be from the food we eat which can be moved directly into working cells or stored as fat. Here again hormones control the situation. For example, insulin is essential for enabling glucose to get into muscle and liver cells. This is the hormone which diabetics lack; there will be more information about this in Chapter 11.

The fuel supply may be assured but it will be of limited value without oxygen. Muscle cells have a small store of oxygen bound to myoglobin (a protein similar to the oxygen-carrying haemoglobin in red blood cells) but this is enough only for about 10 seconds of strenuous work. The muscles are thus dependent for continuing activity upon a more-or-less continuous supply of oxygen from the lungs carried via the bloodstream and propelled by the pumping of the heart. The oxygen is carried partly as dissolved gas but mainly in an easily reversible chemical association with haemoglobin.

Breathing

Breathing movements achieve a tidal flow of air which allows a continuous transport of oxygen through the lungs into the bloodstream and of carbon dioxide in the opposite direction from the bloodstream into the lungs. The lungs and the chest together are like a bellows which is permanently half open. The bony rib cage and the diaphragm form the walls and the floor of a space within the chest and the lungs hang in that space, filling it and adhering to its inner surface by the tension in a thin layer of water. When a person breathes in, the muscular effort enlarges the chest cavity, stretching and expanding the thin elastic lungs so that more air is drawn into them as into a bellows. Breathing out again can be achieved without further muscular effort during quiet respiration because the energy stored in the elastic stretch of the lungs is sufficient to push this air out again. The elastic recoil restores the status quo and the chest cavity becomes smaller again. Extra muscular effort is required to drive the air out when breathing is increased as it is in exercise.

'Breathe in' people say when packing themselves into tight places, or trying to achieve a tiny waist. Breathing in is often confused with pulling the tummy in which results in pushing the air into the top of the chest. Try it.

No amount of muscular effort can completely empty the lungs. About a litre of air (1¾ pints) always remains, so the air brought in with each new breath is mixed with air remaining from the last breath. This has exchanged some of its oxygen for carbon dioxide with the blood passing through the lungs. However hard you breathe you will never quite get the air in your lungs to match the air in the room. Indeed it will make you feel ill if you try, because the carbon dioxide will be removed faster than necessary. Carbon dioxide is important in the control of blood flow to the brain and also of the acidity of the blood. It is therefore essential that its concentration remains within strict limits. Overbreathing does not, on the other hand, significantly increase the amount of oxygen in the blood leaving the lungs because it is already almost fully saturated and so can carry hardly any more.

It is not surprising then that carbon dioxide is a prime regulator of breathing. Blood levels of carbon dioxide influence those nerve cells in the brain which control respiratory movements. If there is a rise in the levels of carbon dioxide in the blood it becomes slightly more acid and this stimulates the respiratory nerve cells into greater activity, and respiratory movements increase in depth and frequency to increase ventilation so that carbon dioxide is carried out of the lungs faster and blood levels fall towards normal. This is one example of a negative feedback loop. Many body systems are controlled by such loops and the effect of this one is to link ventilation to the rate of energy production of the body (metabolic rate).

Ventilation in a theatre or lecture hall must be adequate to remove the waste carbon dioxide produced by its occupants. It is the same with the body but no lecture theatre, even the most modern, can compete with the human body in the elegance of its control of ventilation.

During exercise, ventilation can increase enormously. Brisk walking can send it up from 10 litres (2 gallons) per minute to 60 litres (12 gallons) per minute. In this situation the control system just described is largely overridden by powerful influences exerted by other groups of nerve cells concerned with organizing an adequate total body response to the demands of exercise. This ensures that all parts of the lung are well ventilated, that arterial oxygen will be maintained at a normal level, and that carbon dioxide will be removed fast enough. This happens with time to spare even though the red blood cells spend only a quarter of a second in that part of the lung capillary in which oxygen and carbon dioxide can diffuse freely. The lungs are capable of transferring so much oxygen and carbon dioxide so fast that their function does not limit exercise in normal young individuals.

The situation is quite different in the elderly or the bronchitic. In individuals suffering from chronic lung diseases and asthma the muscular effort of breathing is much increased because the airways are narrowed and impose increased resistance to the flow of air through them; the effort of breathing therefore becomes a limiting factor in oxygen uptake. Such people rapidly become breathless even when walking because they cannot get enough oxygen into their systems to supply the working muscles. The elderly, even if they are free from any insidious lung diseases, have lungs which, like the skin, have lost some of their elasticity. The recoil energy which they can store is therefore less, so the air comes out more slowly and more of it is left behind in the bellows.

The circulation

The capacities of the circulation to transport oxygen and of the muscle cells to extract the oxygen from the blood supplied are all important in exercise. These two factors probably represent those which finally limit the maximum amount of exercise which an individual may take.

The amount of oxygen which gets to the muscle cells will depend upon the amount of blood which is available to flow through the muscle, the quantity of oxygen that the blood can carry, and the proportion of that oxygen which the muscle cells can extract.

The oxygen-carrying capacity of the blood is affected by the amount of haemoglobin in it. In anaemia either the number of red cells or the haemoglobin content of these cells is below normal. This is why capacity for exercise is low in anaemic people and why they are easily tired.

Moving from sea-level to high altitude stimulates an increase in red cell production. At sea-level the air pressure is 760 millimetres of mercury but at 2,500 metres (8,000 feet) the air pressure has dropped to 420 millimetres so the pressure of oxygen is too low to load to capacity the arterial blood leaving the lungs. The only way to restore the oxygen-carrying capacity of the circulation is to increase the number of red blood cells and thus the amount of oxygen that can be carried by each cubic centimetre of blood. This is one of the changes which happens during acclimatization at altitude and why exertion becomes less distressing after two or three weeks.

The need for a big increase in flow of blood through the circulation during exercise is created by the needs of the muscle cells for more oxygen. The accumulation of waste products emerging from the same working cells also needs to be carried away.

The blood flow to the muscles will be dependent upon the output from the heart (cardiac output) and the needs of other tissues. The heart's output in turn depends upon how fast the heart can beat and how big a volume it can pump out at each beat (the stroke volume). Maximum heart rate in children can be over 200 beats a minute, in young adults it rarely exceeds 190 beats a minute, and in older people the limit is about 170. The stroke volume is about 70 millilitres (1 millilitre = 1 cubic centimetre) at rest and it rises even in moderate exercise to near its maximum value of about 120 millilitres.

The cardiac output can increase in several ways, all of which play a part in exercise. The heart is capable of beating steadily without any stimulation but at a rather slow rate, perhaps only 45 or 50 beats per minute. If you count your pulse when you first wake up in the morning before you get out of bed, you will find that it is beating at 60 or 70 beats per minute. So even at rest it is being driven at a faster rate than it could achieve on its own. This is because of the sympathetic accelerator nerves whose activity increases both heart rate and stroke volume. Where there is an accelerator there is normally a brake. In the heart this is provided by the parasympathetic nerves whose activity slows the heart and reduces stroke volume. Groups of nerve cells in the brain which control these nerves constantly adjust the heart rate with a suitable mixture of brake and accelerator.

In addition to all this, adrenalin released into the bloodstream as a circulating hormone has the same effect on the heart as the sympathetic nerves.

A major influence on the heart's output is the amount of blood which returns to it (the venous return). This is so obvious that it escapes most people's notice. If no blood gets back to the heart from the rest of the circulation then there can be no cardiac output at all. If, on the other hand, the venous return is increased then there will be an unwelcome engorgement of the great veins near the heart unless the heart can also increase its output to match. In exercise there is an increased blood flow through working muscles and the rhythmic contraction of those muscles pumps the blood back to the heart through the veins increasing the venous return. The veins have valves which ensure that there is no backflow, so the heart must accommodate the extra blood flow and behave as a pump with a variable stroke. If the heart muscle is stretched by extra blood flowing into it at a slightly higher pressure then it contracts more powerfully owing to the increased stretch. Thus it achieves a bigger stroke volume and a higher output. This ensures that the heart will pump onwards whatever it receives so that in healthy people there is never an embarrassing back pressure in the circulation. In patients with heart failure whose heart muscle is too weak to pump adequately the veins in the neck can be seen bulging with blood which is waiting to be pumped round.

Because of the stretching effect of returning blood, normal hearts can deal satisfactorily with an increased venous return and turn it into an increased cardiac output but there is nothing they can do about a reduced venous return. The effects of gravity on the blood in the legs is sometimes enough to reduce venous return and therefore cardiac output to such low levels that the brain does not get enough blood and the person faints. This sometimes happens when people stand up quickly or to Guardsmen standing still on parade for a long time in hot weather. Once on the floor in a horizontal position the circulation is restored and the person recovers. Never try to prop up a fainting person.

During exercise because of the increased cardiac output it is normal for the arterial blood pressure to increase. The increased head of pressure ensures the necessary large increase in muscle blood flow without prejudicing flow to other essential places like the brain sited as it is in a vulnerable position above the pump. In vigorous exercise the increase may amount to almost a doubling of the peak pressure (systolic, while the heart is expelling the blood). The trough pressure (diastolic, between beats) does not change appreciably. The difference between peak and trough can be detected in large arteries at the wrist or neck as a pulse, which feels more forceful just after exercise than at rest. Once the blood has reached the small capillaries where the oxygen is given up the flow is smooth.

The increase in total flow produced by the heart is shared by the contracting muscles, the heart itself, and the skin. Distribution of flow is achieved by dilating or constricting the appropriate net-works of blood-vessels. The increase in blood flow through the skin is required to dissipate the heat produced in the muscles. The blood flow to the brain is unchanged. Some of the blood which flows through the muscle has been diverted from the intestines and kidneys. This is why it is unwise to exercise vigorously after a big meal. In this situation there is not enough blood to go round so there are distribution problems and priority decisions have to be made. In intense exercise blood flow may be diverted away from the skin despite increasing deep body temperature. Temperature regulation is temporarily sacrificed for the sake of the working muscles. During a game of squash the skin may be pale, but at the end of the game the skin flushes pink and the players feel hotter but also more comfortable. They can now get rid of their heat load freely once the muscles are no longer making such big demands on blood flow.

Waste disposal

If the air is cooler than the core of the body then heat will be steadily transferred from the body surface to the air. Air currents and wind further increase heat loss. A brisk walker can, by removing the insulating layers provided by a jumper or a coat, achieve a comfortable equilibrium between heat produced and heat lost, so can someone running out of doors in cold weather. In a warm environment something more is needed, and the main heat loss is through an increased blood flow to the skin allowing both improved direct losses to the air as well as loss by sweating. The liquid sweat removes heat as it turns into water vapour and drifts away.

These responses are highly effective in preventing the temperature deep within the body from rising more than one or two degrees above normal, but they require a substantial share of the total blood flow. Skin blood flow rises from 1 or 2 per cent of total flow to 20 per cent in prolonged heavy exercise, for example digging in warm conditions. This means that the heart must beat faster to maintain the blood flow to the working muscles and explains why hard work in the heat is a greater stress than hard work in the cold.

It is often alleged that hot tea is more refreshing than cold orange squash in hot weather. The apparent paradox arises because the hot tea increases the deep temperature of the body, heat-sensitive cells in the brain detect this and through their controlling nerves increase the activity of the sweat glands. More sweat produces a cooler skin and so the tea drinker feels better although he is temporarily hotter inside. He is more aware of his skin temperature than his deep body temperature.

Water loss through prolonged sweating can amount to many litres. Coal-miners working hard in an enclosed warm environment can lose up to 1½ litres (2½ pints) per hour. There will also be a loss of salt. Since the total blood volume is 5 or 6 litres (9 or 10 pints) a dangerous state of dehydration and heat stroke can develop if the water and salt are not replaced. The miner needs his beer! Water conservation is temporarily sacrificed for the sake of temperature regulation.

Heat can be regarded as a waste product of vigorous exercise. The other product of energy release which must be disposed of rapidly, just as in the central-heating boiler, is carbon dioxide. This is the residue from the complete oxidative breakdown of glucose and fats. It will diffuse out from the working cells into the bloodstream, while the oxygen is diffusing in the opposite direction; it will be carried in the blood to the lungs, mainly in solution and partly in various loose chemical combinations with the protein molecules of the blood; it will then diffuse across the lung capillary wall, across the lung membrane, and out. All the movements of the oxygen and carbon dioxide are by rapid diffusion from areas of higher concentration to areas of lower concentration. This takes place over the very large surface areas of the lung capillaries or the capillary networks of the working muscles. In the lungs these small blood-vessels provide a surface at least as big as a tennis court.

The components of the transport chains for oxygen and carbon dioxide are summarized diagrammatically in Figure 4 (page 20).

Limits

In a healthy person the systems are well tuned, their components matched and integrated, so it is difficult to pin-point with certainty which link in the chain is the weakest. Moreover, the limiting factors may vary from one person to another and within one person from one time to another, depending upon state of health and training.

It seems likely that in normal people the limitations to prolonged strenuous effort with large muscles are set by the rate at which the heart and blood-vessels can deliver oxygen to the muscles. Limits for other kinds of muscular work, such as a short sprint (high

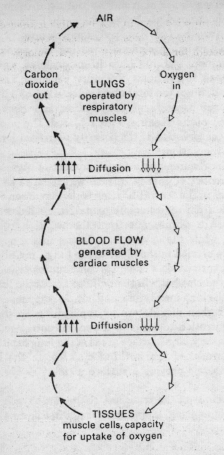

AIR

Carbon dioxide out

LUNGS operated by respiratory muscles

Oxygen in

↑↑↑↑ Diffusion ↓↓↓↓

BLOOD FLOW generated by cardiac muscles

↑↑↑↑ Diffusion ↓↓↓↓

TISSUES muscle cells, capacity for uptake of oxygen

Fig. 4. The transport chains for oxygen and carbon dioxide
Oxygen delivery is only effectively achieved if each link in the chain is adequate

intensity, short duration) or a day's ramble (low intensity, long duration), are quite different. The limits are probably largely in the muscles themselves, and they have a great potential for improvement.

Short and sharp

In a sprint the muscles have to rely heavily on anaerobic (without oxygen available) energy release, because oxygen cannot be delivered fast enough for aerobic (with oxygen) energy sources to be used. Some of the energy stored as glucose can be released by partial breakdown of the glucose to form lactic acid. This happens in the absence of oxygen, hence the term anaerobic. The limit to the intensity of anaerobic exercise is the rate at which the muscle cells can convert the chemical energy from glucose breakdown into the energy of movement. The cardio-vascular system plays no part in this. The duration of high-intensity anaerobic exercise is always short because it is limited by the rising levels of lactic acid and other acidic waste substances. This causes increasing acidity of the blood which leads to powerful stimulation of the respiratory control centres in the brain and increasing breathlessness amounting to extreme respiratory distress. This is why we can sprint over a short distance, to catch a bus or a wayward child, whereas we could not possibly complete a cross-country run at that speed. There is also increasing pain in the active muscles owing to the accumulation of lactic acid and probably other unknown substances released by activity of the muscle cells. If we try sawing up logs, this kind of pain develops in the working arm muscles fairly quickly. Slowing down our rate of sawing is no help because the saw gets stuck in the wood. The only way out is to stop and rest until the pain goes.

The limits we are aware of are aching muscles especially when the small muscles of the arms are used and distressed breathing especially when the large leg muscles are used. This happens because the muscles are struggling to mobilize energy without being able to take up oxygen and lose waste substances fast enough, and because the breathing is being overdriven by the acids released from muscles mobilizing energy without enough oxygen. Some people are also aware of their heart pounding away in their chest. In practice only youngsters and athletes exercise long enough and hard enough to drive their heart rate up to its maximum. The aching legs and uncomfortable breathing can be regarded as providing a wide safety margin which protects the whole system from damage.

Slow and steady

Over long distances the cardio-respiratory (heart-lung) system is fully capable of maintaining the oxygen supply needed for the moderate exercise involved. After a walk of several hours most people retire with vague feelings of fatigue which are enjoyable rather than unpleasant, or at the worst some blisters on their feet. Under more unusual circumstances, say an army route march in a hot climate, collapse can occur for a number of reasons. Glucose supplies may become exhausted and then fatty acids are processed abnormally in the cells to form acidic substances. Dehydration may occur as a result of the sweating needed to contain the rising body temperature. Dehydration can lead to changes in the concentration of salts in the body which can cause malfunction of the heart and nervous system. These things can also happen in marathon runs, but few people ever reach such extremes of exhaustion.

Hold it!

The limits for maintained muscular effort, such as holding up a shelf, pushing a car, or carrying a heavy suitcase, are different again. This is because instead of working by intermittently contracting and relaxing, as in running, the muscles are in a state of continuous contraction, which impedes their blood supply. The cardio-vascular control system in the brain responds by rapidly increasing the heart rate and the blood pressure. This can be seen as a futile attempt to perfuse the tightly contracted muscle. This kind of muscular activity is always short lived if the contraction is at more than 15 per cent of the muscle's maximum strength, because the accumulation of waste products in the active muscle causes increasing pain and finally sudden failure of contraction. As soon as the muscle relaxes blood flow is restored and recovery is rapid. If carried to extremes, this kind of maintained exercise is probably the most dangerous kind of exercise for older people that they are likely to encounter in daily living, not because of danger to the muscles but because a steep rise in blood pressure may place a strain on any weaknesses in blood-vessels. If the weakness is in a blood-vessel supplying the brain there is the possibility of a cerebral haemorrhage (stroke). It also increases the work-load of the heart giving rise to angina (chest pain) in susceptible people.

Recovery

Recovery from short bouts of exercise takes only a few minutes, recovery from prolonged strenuous exercise sometimes takes many hours. It will be clear from the foregoing descriptions that widespread changes can occur and that the nature and degree of these changes vary according to the kind of exercise.

In rhythmic moderate exercise, such as walking or ballroom dancing, a steady state is attained which can last for long periods. After such exercise, the heart rate, ventilation rate, and muscle blood flow drop rapidly and within a few minutes they will have returned to near resting levels. The heart rate and cardiac output may remain slightly elevated for 15 to 20 minutes while the rate of heat loss returns to normal. There is a lag due to the storage of heat in the body. One of the most notable subjective after-effects of any exercise is the sudden feeling of warmth which occurs when movement stops and there is no longer a flow of air removing body heat. Restoration of stores of muscle glycogen (polyglucose) will take place later after some carbohydrate food has been eaten and will take several hours.

Rhythmic exercise of high intensity and short duration, such as the fathers' race on sports' day, produces greater immediate changes and a longer recovery period. Heart rate, ventilation rate, and muscle blood flow may take many minutes to return to normal. Because the exercise is of high intensity the energy release will have been largely anaerobic. The aftermath is an accumulation of lactic acid, other waste products of exercise, and an oxygen 'debt'. The oxygen 'debt' is the amount of oxygen which would have been used if the same amount of energy had been expended over a longer time span. It is needed after intense exercise to 'pay back' muscle stores and to complete the breakdown of lactic acid to glucose. This releases further energy which can be stored. A maintained muscle blood flow is needed for a short time to flush out the other accumulated products of energy release. There will be a lag in the dissipation of heat as in moderate exercise, and a further amount of heat will be released during the energy transactions involved in repayment of the oxygen debt. The longer and more intense this exercise is, the greater the oxygen debt and the longer the recovery period. As before there is a need to replace glycogen stores, which will take several hours.

The after-effects of maintained muscle contraction are short lived. There is a transient increase in muscle blood flow which washes out the accumulated waste products, and the heart rate and blood pressure return rapidly to normal.

Fatigue

The stiffness which is commonly observed after unaccustomed severe exercise is thought to be due to minor injury and swelling. It is cured by a judicious mixture of rest and further exercise and results in stronger muscles. The magical effects of a hot bath may be due to increased muscle blood flow washing out pain-stimulating products of tissue damage or to the relaxation induced. Cramp is sometimes due to muscle spasm brought on by changes in the concentrations of certain salts in the fluid bathing the muscle cells which make the muscle more sensitive and therefore more liable to contract. It can also be caused by the stimulus of intense cold which may occur during swimming in the sea. Cramp is painful because, by contracting, the muscle compresses the blood-vessels within it, severely limiting its own blood supply in just the same way as with a maintained contraction.

Stiffness, cramp, and fatigue are all ill understood. Muscle fatigue must be defined as failure to generate force. This can happen as a result of failure at any one of a number of links in the chain. Muscle contraction is initiated by nerve cells in the brain, some of them at conscious levels, some of them subconscious. Learning to ride a bicycle, swim, or drive a car involves consciously controlled movements at first. Later these movements become automatic and are initiated from subconscious brain centres. The messages from the brain are relayed through the telegraphic system of the nerves through connections in the spinal cord and eventually through motor nerves to the muscles. The message must get across the nerve–muscle junction by the release of small packets of a chemical substance which diffuse across the gap and stimulate the muscle membrane into activity. This in turn sets off a sequence of events consisting mainly of chemical reactions leading to the breakdown of ATP to release energy which can then be used by the muscle cell in order to contract.

There are many diseases in which the links in this long chain are broken. Strokes can leave people paralysed because the brain cells initiating movement have died; poliomyelitis paralyses because it destroys the nerve cells of the spinal cord which control muscle contraction. After long disuse, for example when a limb is in a plaster cast because of broken bones, the muscles literally drop out of mind. The brain no longer 'remembers' that they exist. It can be 'reminded' by directly stimulating the muscle membrane with a small electric current. The muscle contracts and this sets off streams of information which are carried back through nerve pathways to the brain from the muscle. The ability to initiate the muscle contraction voluntarily is then restored.

This is not, however, what is meant by fatigue. In normal people it usually occurs in the muscle cell itself when it runs out of energy supplies. This happens relatively quickly in maintained contractions and in intense bursts of intermittent exercise. The ATP supplies fail because the by-products of energy released in the absence of enough oxygen are sufficient to inhibit further release of energy from glucose. In practice the discomfort produced in muscles which are obliged to work anaerobically is enough to prevent people from continuing the exercise to its physiological limit.

Fatigue is a subjective matter and has a large psychological component as well as various physical bases. Symptoms can be overridden if motivation is powerful enough. If a large sum of money is offered, the pain will be endured and the muscles previously declared to be totally fatigued will continue to contract. Fear as well as financial inducement will do the trick. There is a tale of a man who jumped over a wall while being chased by a bull. Later when the bull had gone he was quite unable to jump back over the wall.

Fatigue after long periods of mild exercise is less well understood. It is partly a matter of boredom. There is a need for variety in activity. There is also a need for sleep which still baffles those who try to find out why that should be so.

2

THE EFFECTS OF TRAINING

You can't put it in the bank

Muscles need to be kept in training. If they are not used their capacity for doing their job deteriorates. Fortunately for us this deterioration is not irreversible like the rusting up of machinery. Muscle cells shrink and become weaker with lack of use, but they always retain their capacity for growing larger and stronger again with appropriate exercise.

Many body systems can to some extent adapt to increased demands with an improved performance and conversely the performance will dwindle if it is seldom or never called forth. Muscles have this adaptability to a marked degree. Although in the end our maximum capacities for physical work are limited by body size and proportion, which are in turn largely genetically determined, the degree to which we realize our potential within those limits depends upon how much and in what ways we use our muscles.

If we take little exercise our muscle strength and capacity for prolonged physical exertion are probably at about half their potential value. However, if we then begin to make more use of our muscles on a regular basis they can do more work and work for longer without protest. This process of improving muscle strength and capacity for work by increasing exercise levels is what is meant by training.

It does not require endless strenuous 'work-outs' except for those who are already athletic. The important thing is to do a little more than normal. If you drive a car to the office where you sit at a desk until it is time to drive home and put your feet up, then a brisk walk for half an hour three times a week will work wonders. You will feel a new person because of the changes induced by training. Those who start off from the worst position with a recent record of almost no physical activity will find it easiest to improve. If you are at the bottom of the pile, there is nowhere to go except up, whereas for those in good shape training is arduous. This is the principle of overload; training is only produced by an *increase* in physical activity. Walking will only produce improvements in those who previously took very little exercise; if you are already used to running then walking will not train you.

The effects of the extra exercise are cumulative and take time to develop. A sudden single bout of strenuous exercise will produce only stiffness, and if there are any training effects they will be too transient to be noticeable. So the extra exercise must be continued, not necessarily with rigid regularity, but at least at intervals of a few days. Badminton several times a week would qualify, so would walking up to the fifth floor every day instead of taking the lift.

Unfortunately, the improvements disappear again over a period of weeks if exercise levels are allowed to fall. This is the next general principle of training, that you cannot put it in the bank. However, the improvements can be maintained by less exercise than was required to achieve them in the first place. The investment only becomes worthless if you forget to pay your instalments.

Any physical activity which involves the generation of force by muscles can be considered exercise. There is the physical activity of the job including the effort of getting there, active leisure pursuits like swimming, rambling, or old-time dancing, and of course deliberate exercise like jogging or keep fit classes. Any increase in daily exercise level can produce improvement in the way the body adapts to exercise, and then the exercise feels easier. Training is the process of producing that improvement.

However, since different types of exercise have different effects on body systems, as was explained in Chapter 1, it is not surprising that training effects also differ according to the type of exercise. This is the third principle of training. Its effects are specific for the kind of exercise and the muscles used. Muscle strength, the flexibility of joints (range of movements), skill (the co-ordination of movements), and stamina (the capacity for rhythmic exercise) can all be improved with the right kind of exercise. These different aspects of fitness for physical activity will be discussed in turn, but first of all, why is training so specific?

The main effects of training are on the working muscles of the limbs and not on the heart and lungs as many people think. This is why training effects are specific to the muscles used. Running will not improve your capacity for rowing very much. Moreover, training is also specific to the kind of exercise. Weight-lifting or short, sharp bouts of exercise increase muscle strength but do not improve stamina. Endurance exercise such as walking for hours improves stamina but not muscle strength. The reason is that there are two kinds of muscle cell which are differentially affected. The fast-twitch muscle cells, as their name implies, are used for short, sharp bursts of activity and can work anaerobically (without oxygen) whereas the slow-twitch fibres have a high capacity for taking up and using oxygen, and are best suited to endurance activities. These differences have only recently been discovered. Research techniques developed in Scandinavia have made it possible to look at small cores of muscle tissue, analyse the contents of the cells, and discover a great deal more about what is going on inside them. This is a technique known as muscle biopsy.

The fast muscle cells are pale in colour and rich in the enzymes which control rapid energy release in the absence of oxygen. Fast muscle cells can release energy at six times the rate of the so-called slow ones. They are predominantly used for the short, sharp kinds of physical effort in which oxygen supplies are restricted. This includes maintained exercise when the oxygen supply to the muscle is blocked by its own contraction. Also high-intensity rhythmic exercise like running upstairs when there is not enough time for an adequate oxygen delivery.

The slow muscle cells are red in colour because they are rich in myoglobin which, like its close relation haemoglobin, stores oxygen. They are also packed with enzymes concerned with the release of energy from oxygen and energy stores. They are used predominantly for the maintenance of posture and for endurance exercise such as walking or cycling which must depend on a steady oxygen supply. They are for stamina. Long-distance runners, for instance, have a high proportion of slow muscle cells. In some countries muscle biopsies are used to predict the events in which aspiring young athletes are likely to excel. The sport that you choose or the exercise pattern you adopt is likely to be influenced by the proportions of muscle cells with which you happen to have been born.

Maintained exercise or high-intensity activity of short duration will train the fast muscle cells and have little or no effect on the slow ones whereas rhythmic exercise will train the oxidative enzymes in both slow and fast muscle cells. This is why training is specific not only to the muscles used but also to the kind of exercise. There are racing cyclists who can clock up record times for 100-mile rides but put them on the ground to walk and half an hour's shopping exhaust them, whereas the housewives or shop assistants who are on their feet all day wouldn't last ten minutes on a bicycle.

If you want to become better at doing something then practise that something. If you want to be able to swim for twenty minutes without stopping and justify your continued ownership of the

Fig. 5. Changes in a muscle cell after training

Change	Effect
More muscle protein	Greater muscle strength
More enzymes for energy release without oxygen	Faster performance in short intense exercise
More enzymes releasing energy using oxygen More capillary blood-vessels bringing oxygen	Improved stamina

bronze medal you earned at school, then practise swimming. Sprinting or weight-lifting would help the swimming a little in that they strengthen the muscles of the arms and legs but the effects would be marginal.

The three principles of training
The worse you are the easier it is to improve
It doesn't last
It is specific to the muscles used

Muscle strength

Maintained exercise, also called static exercise or isometrics, will increase muscle strength if the exercise is intense enough. It doesn't matter if the muscle contraction is maintained for a very short time, indeed it should be short otherwise it gives rise to large increases in blood pressure. The crucial requirement is that the intensity of the contraction must be over 80 per cent of the muscle's own maximum strength.

For example, squeezing a tennis ball hard for a couple of seconds many times a day will increase the strength of the arm muscles responsible for flexing the fingers in a 'power' grip. The ball can live in a pocket and no one will know about the training until they shake hands with you in a few weeks' time. After that you will be in perpetual demand for getting recalcitrant lids off screw-top jars.

Training is specific to the muscles used. Squeezing a tennis ball will obviously do nothing for the strength of the leg muscles. So a variety of exercises or activities are needed if you want to keep all the muscles in good trim. Keep fit classes and books of exercises aim to help you to do just that.

It is of especial importance to maintain the muscles of the trunk, both back and abdomen, because these provide a stable foundation against which the limb muscles can work. This becomes apparent when unaccustomed activity, whether it be wind-surfing, gardening, or just an unusually long walk, leaves a slight feeling of stiffness in many trunk muscles as well as in the leg or arm muscles which have had to work harder than normal.

Many yoga exercises will strengthen trunk muscles but they must be performed without strain so that improvement is gradual. Damage can be done by putting too much tension on weak ligaments which are not protected by adequately strong muscles.

Strength training using maintained contraction is effective because it eventually increases the amount of specialized protein in the fast muscle cells. It is this protein which allows the muscles to pull. Eating more meat will not increase your own muscle protein. It will be turned into fat or glucose unless strength training provides the stimulus for your muscle cells to remake it into their own muscle protein. Strength training also increases the concentration of those enzymes responsible for energy release without oxygen. It is the kind of training practised by weight-lifters who do so much that the increase in contractile protein becomes apparent as a noticeable increase in muscle size. However, it is not necessary to develop bulging muscles in order to increase muscle strength. Lifting a heavy teapot will become easier long before bulging biceps become apparent. This kind of training also increases the strength of tendons and ligaments so that they can withstand the increased pull of the muscles.

Flexibility of joints

Yoga exercises and some of the keep fit exercises are intended to maintain or achieve the full range of movement of joints. This is important because joints stiffen up with disuse. Again caution is necessary. Improvements should be gradual and never taken to extremes. It is possible to make joints so flexible that they lose stability, and become liable to dislocate. Muscles as well as ligaments are essential for stabilizing joints and preventing the dislocations which can happen with a sudden load. So a happy medium of flexibility is required, coupled with a safety margin of strength in the muscles.

An arm or leg that has been incarcerated in a plaster cast because of broken bones emerges from its cocoon with limited movement and weak muscles. The continual wearing of high heels can lead to a shortening of the Achilles tendon at the back of the heel and a restriction in the range of ankle movement. It has been known for women to break their Achilles tendon in their efforts to get fit. This can happen if they change their high heels for flat plimsolls and then jump down the steps. The muscle is shorter and can no longer operate as a shock absorber, the tendon proves to be the weak link and breaks when they land. What is needed in both these situations is a gentle stretching of the shortened muscles and, for recovery after having a limb in plaster, the redevelopment of muscle strength.

Swimming is an excellent kind of exercise for restoring or maintaining strength and mobility, because it does not involve weight-bearing. In the swimming-pool the water takes the weight and all movements are cushioned. This means that excessive strains on weak joints and muscles will be avoided. The maximum force that can be applied to the joint is not more than its own muscles can muster. The effects of gravity have been removed.

Skill

The rule that benefits gained by training for one activity cannot be transferred to another also extends to the development of skill and co-ordination. The first stages of learning to drive, swim, or ride a bicycle are clumsy and only achieved at all by concentrated mental effort. Practice eventually results in smooth effective movements and appropriate postural balance. The kangaroo juice disappears from the petrol tank, a length of the swimming pool is achieved without panic, and the wayward bicycle no longer has a mind of its own. Control has been achieved. This happens as the co-ordinating nerve pathways are established in subconscious areas of the brain and conscious control is no longer necessary. The necessary muscle strength will usually develop at the same time. This is achieved only through repeated effort and there is no transfer of skill between different activities.

It is obvious that the patterning of movements is unique to each activity and yet it is a common observation that sportsmen are often good at many sports rather than just one. There are two reasons for this. One is that there are common elements in sports, for instance the hand–eye co-ordination needed to hit a ball with a bat. The other reason may be that potential sportsmen are born with a plentiful supply of the appropriate nerve pathways, and so have a latent ability for good motor co-ordination which will require a minimum of training. They will take to ball games like ducks to water.

Stamina

Rhythmic exercise of moderate intensity which can be maintained for half an hour or more is often called endurance exercise. It has quite different effects from maintained muscle contractions or the short, sharp bouts of exercise which improve muscle strength. Endurance exercise like walking, jogging, swimming, or cycling improves stamina and endurance because it increases the capacity for taking up and using oxygen, so aerobic exercise can be sustained at a higher intensity and for longer.

Again the main changes are in the muscles, this time in the slow muscle cells and also to some extent in the circulatory system. Lung function is not altered by any form of training and does not limit aerobic exercise in healthy people.

The slow muscle cells respond to endurance training by manufacturing higher concentrations of enzymes for handling oxygen and the oxidative release of energy from glucose and fats. They are therefore better equipped to take up and use the oxygen being supplied to them in the bloodstream. This improvement is further enhanced by the growth of a more abundant capillary network. Each muscle cell is now nearer to a blood-borne source of oxygen and nutrients. Because of these changes their maximum capacity for aerobic energy release is increased; stamina and endurance improve.

The muscle will be able to work harder using oxidative energy sources only. It will not need to rely on anaerobic energy supplies until the work intensity is much higher. Capacity for endurance exercise therefore goes up. Brisk walking can now be maintained indefinitely whereas previously anything faster than 5 kilometres per hour (3 mph) produced a slowing-down within minutes due to increasing breathlessness and protesting muscles.

Also, at lower than maximum rates of work the muscle can manage on a smaller blood flow because it can extract more oxygen from each passing drop of blood. A further result of this improved oxidative capacity and consequent reduction in blood flow is that the working muscle makes smaller demands on the circulation as a whole and blood flow to the other areas like the skin or the digestive tract will be less restricted.

Endurance exercise trains not only the muscle cells but also the circulatory system. There are two ways in which the circulation can be affected, one is direct and the other is a consequence of the changes in the muscles.

The direct effects are an increase in the strength of contraction of the heart which results in a larger stroke volume and a larger maximum output. The pump empties itself more completely and is therefore more effective. Also there is a small increase in blood volume which makes more blood available to meet the various competing demands during exercise.

One of the reasons why a week in bed leaves the victim feeling so debilitated is the reduction in blood volume which happens after lying flat for several days. Much less fluid is needed in the blood-vessels to maintain an adequate circulation in this position, but, once upright again, man is vulnerable to the effects of gravity. The veins can behave like large elastic reservoirs in which the blood collects under the influence of gravity. This can leave the pumping heart with too little blood returning to it. Despite its best effort there is no way it can maintain enough pressure for blood to flow up to the brain. Temporary loss of consciousness inevitably follows. This is what happens during a faint. As soon as the horizontal position is regained, blood flow is restored to the brain and consciousness returns. It would be dangerous to prop the victim up. So blood volume is important, but the changes which follow from the improved capacity of the muscle cells to take up and use oxygen are even more important.

Perhaps because of changes in the demands of the muscles for blood flow the response of the heart to exercise changes. Heart rate always goes up in response to exercise to meet the need for increased flow without losing any driving pressure. After training with endurance exercise, the heart rate rises much less although the total flow (cardiac output) is unchanged. This must mean that there is an increase in stroke volume if the same cardiac output is to be maintained with a lower heart rate. The consequence of this is that the heart has less work to do in order to achieve the same cardiac output. It is more economical for the pump to work slowly with a large stroke rather than fast and with a small stroke. There is an improvement both in the way the pump works and in the way its output is distributed.

Endurance exercise therefore improves both the working muscles and the economy of the circulation. The net result of all these changes is that any given physical task can be achieved with less strain. It feels less tiring, less of a burden because the muscles are using a smaller proportion of their maximum ability and the heart rate is much lower.

The next question is how much extra endurance exercise is needed to produce noticeable improvements, how hard must the exercise be, for how long should we do it, and how often must it be repeated?

The effects of endurance training can be dramatic. Improvements of 30 per cent in maximal energy output have been observed in a small group of young men who increased their exercise levels as much as possible by first resting in bed for several weeks and then embarking on strenuous training. Numerous other studies have shown that any increase in the intensity of physical activity improves the capacity for that activity. This is true for anyone, regardless of age, sex, or level of physical ability, with the exception of athletes in training who may have reached their genetically limited potential.

How can the improvements best be achieved, and what is the right dose of exercise? It is not possible to draw up specific prescriptions, each individual must feel his way to his own right dose because he is the only one who has full access to his previous history and all the hints he gets from his own protesting joints, aching muscles, thumping heart, or bursting lungs. Nevertheless, some clear guidelines have been established.

How much exercise for improvements in stamina?

How hard? A little harder or faster than is customary for you

How often? Three times a week

How long for? Twenty minutes

The watchword is to increase the amount and intensity of the exercise slowly; start from what you know you can do, and then go a little further or a little faster each time, being patient with yourself.

Marked improvements can be achieved with walking if you are not used to exercise. If your exercise leaves you red-faced and speechless at the time, and stiff the next day, then it is too strenuous. When you can't walk any faster and you don't want to walk any further because you have already been walking for hours and it's taking up too much time, then jog. The change-over comes at about 7 kilometres per hour (4¼ mph). Start with a combination of two minutes' jogging (slow running) and two minutes' walking and gradually lengthen the contribution made by the jogging as the days pass by.

Intermittent rests are essential at the beginning, always start with a 'warm-up' and finish gradually with a 'warm-down'; in other words, don't start and stop vigorous exercise suddenly. Remember that 80 per cent of your energy expenditure is going to be released as heat so wear sensible clothes that are loose, comfortable, and cool. Mechanical damage to the feet is common at the start of an exercise programme so wear purpose-built shoes which fit, are comfortable, and stay on! This means walking shoes, plimsolls, or running shoes, all of which have laces for proper fit round the instep.

The effects of innumerable different training schemes on large numbers of people have been measured and the consensus of opinion is that twenty to thirty minutes of extra exercise three times a week is the minimum required to produce improvements; a little less than that will maintain them. One study has shown that three times a week is as good if not better than five times for improving capacity for exercise.

You can work harder
for longer
with less effort

The effects of the exercise will depend upon its intensity, duration, and frequency provided that the dose has not been so high that it has caused excessive stiffness or damage. An encouraging message for the unfit and poorly motivated is that the worse you are the easier it is to improve. Age is no barrier to training provided you start from where you are now and increase the dose gradually. It is what you did yesterday that counts; so if you have been desk-bound in recent years, then it is irrelevant that you were once the school's champion runner. Similarly, if you are ill in bed, or lapse from a training programme, your physical condition will deteriorate and it will be necessary to reduce your training level to avoid excessive strain and fatigue. Unfortunately, training is reversible. It is possible to acquire good physical condition, with an effort, but it cannot then be put into storage, it must be used or it will be lost again.

It seems likely that increases in customary levels of activity, whether achieved by a deliberate training programme or a more active job, set off a positive feedback cycle in which the improved exercise capacity leads to even more physical activity. The exercise becomes self-reinforcing. Unfortunately, the converse is likely to happen as well, that lack of exercise leads to a deterioration in physical condition and to less exercise. Is it possible to maintain an equilibrium between two such spirals? The best solution is surely to retain a capacity for exercise which is compatible with one's life-style and still allows a wide choice of possible physical activities.

Fortunately, even after many years of inactivity muscle strength and stamina can be regained, but the cure is not obtainable on prescription or by special dieting, the only way is to take more exercise and to do so regularly.

This is comforting knowledge; even if you are flabby and middle-aged you can take heart. The investment of a little more physical effort at intervals will be rewarded by the ability to work with less physical effort whenever you have a need. This is a paradox which none of us should neglect.

An increased capacity for physical activity often leads to a renewed *joie de vivre*, new possibilities in daily life may open up, and far-reaching psychological benefits may follow.

All this would seem justification enough for the promotion of exercise as one of the good things in life, regardless of its possible curative or protective effects in disease. Moreover, unlike most of the good things in life, it can be free.

3

CHILDREN AND EXERCISE

Games should be fun

Young children are spontaneously active, sometimes so much so that their parents and relations complain and say that they feel tired just looking at them. This is a sober reflection on how far the adults have let their physical resources deteriorate, not an indictment of the children. They can be seen any day of the week running round the school playgrounds, playing games of catch, kicking a ball, or thumping each other enthusiastically, whereas the typical adolescent 'hangs round' in a group just talking in a desultory manner. This impression has been confirmed by a few studies in which it has been found that only about a quarter of 13-, 14- and 15-year-old boys engage in vigorous activity.

The important question is whether exercise or lack of it influences the development or growth of young children or adolescents. It is possible that television, high-rise flats, and the motor car are contributing to a big drop in the activity levels of some children. If they become absorbed in television for many hours a day, then there is little time left for more energetic pleasures. High-rise flats provide no space for children who want to play physically demanding games. To their parents television appears to be safer than playing in the streets but in the long run too much of it may be an insidious threat to health by displacing active play. More families than ever before possess a car so children ride in them to school and elsewhere instead of managing on foot or on a bicycle.

Reliable assessments are hard to find but there is a growing suspicion that even young children may be less physically active than they were twenty years ago. If this is so then two questions arise. Will reduced activity levels unfavourably influence growth and development, and will an inactive life-style in childhood make it even more difficult to maintain levels of activity comparable with optimum health in adult life?

These are hard questions to answer. The second one is a matter for speculation and will probably remain so, because measuring levels of habitual daily activity is difficult and most research workers are daunted by the prospect of mounting a study which would last for twenty years or more.

Attempts have been made to answer the first question. Illness and the inevitable inactivity associated with it slow down a child's rate of growth. This may be due more to the illness than to the lack of exercise and in any case, once recovered from the disease, the child appears to catch up if given time. Growth will go on into the late teens and early twenties in children whose adolescence has been disturbed by illness.

Nevertheless an uneasy suspicion remains that a continuous restriction of physical scope all through the growing years may have permanent consequences. In support of this there is one study in which smaller lung size in children has been found in association with cramped housing. There may be a threshold level for activity which must be achieved if the full potential of a child's genetic endowment is to find expression in his adult size.

If we now consider vigorous exercise rather than inadequate activity, is there any evidence that this produces an enhancement of growth and development in children? The strenuous training of adolescent youngsters, for swimming or football for instance, can produce the same improvements as it does in adults. The muscles and circulation can take up more oxygen and performance improves. It is also alleged that athletic training of children or adolescents increases performance in a second more dramatic way by accelerating their growth. Girl swimmers who trained for international competition developed bigger hearts, lungs, muscles, and bones and it was suggested that this would ultimately give them greater adult stature and exercise capacity. This was an exciting possibility. Was a race of super-people possible after all? The critics, however, were quick to point out that the individuals who become élite athletes are well endowed physically in the first place and so are likely to grow tall and strong even without the benefit of swimming for five hours a day for months on end. Furthermore when the training stopped the size of the heart and skeletal muscles decreased again.

The problem with all these claims for both the impairment due to inactivity and the improvement due to training is that it is not possible to predict with any certainty how fast or how big a child will grow. Growth curves are not uniform. Immediately after birth infants grow very quickly, but their speed of growth slows down steadily until they are about 2 or 3 years of age. The average rate of growth of young children over each of the following years then shows a slower steady decrease until adolescence begins. However, within any given year, the growth rate may change dramatically. Some children may scarcely grow at all for a period of three months, and then grow very quickly in the following three months. Any parent trying to keep children respectably clad will appreciate this point.

This slow decline in growth rate over the primary school years is reversed by the onset of the adolescent spurt which is associated with developing sexual maturity. This can happen quite suddenly and at variable and unpredictable ages, any time between 9 and 13 years of age for girls and between 11 and 14 years for boys. Thus if one were to study the apparent effect of exercise on a group of 9-year-old girls, it would appear to accelerate markedly the growth of a few but have no effect at all on most. A similar study of 13-year-olds would indicate that growth was apparently slowed down dramatically by the exercise, while in others the effect would vary from a slight acceleration to a dramatic one. The same argument in relation to strength as well as size can be applied to boys.

The effects of training cannot be clearly separated from the considerable increase in the dimensions of the heart and lungs, together with body size in general, which occur during the adolescent spurt in the absence of training. There is no simple criterion by which suitable 'control' subjects could be selected as being in exactly the same stage of the adolescent spurt as others who were undergoing the training. Thus it is not possible to separate the effects of the training from the considerable increases in exercise capacity which will take place anyway simply as a result of a child's natural growth as determined by his genetic endowment.

Apart from the difficulty of sorting out the permanent effects of deliberate training and spontaneous growth, youngsters do respond to exercise in similar ways to adults. Increased exercise levels will produce improvements and a reduction will result in deterioration. Anyone who has tried training a reluctant secondary school team knows very well that the exercise recipe only works if the children will stick at it; and that the rot sets in all too quickly if they don't. Younger, more lively children are rather different.

They are already so active that training is a matter of developing skills rather than exercise capacity. They already have abundant energy and the practice brings control.

On the other hand, children who are physically or mentally handicapped may drop below the hypothetical exercise threshold. Certainly they are not usually as spontaneously active as their normal peers and unless the adults who care for them organize their physical play activities they may not achieve their optimum development. This is especially important since that optimum may still leave much to be desired.

For the handicapped of any age it is vital to make the most of the function which remains and in children this is so for two reasons. In the first place, because of the suspicion that there is a threshold for optimum growth, and secondly, because even small physical gains may lead to psychological improvements which in turn stimulate physical efforts. Physical achievements make us all feel better, and the handicapped are no exception. The wheelchair Olympics should never be far from the minds of those who shape the aspirations of the young and handicapped. If the sky is the limit there is much more chance of getting off the ground.

Severe obesity in childhood might well be considered a handicap as well as the more obvious ones. It makes osteo-arthritis in later life more likely because the increased body weight may sufficiently change the shape of the thigh bone so that the load on the hips and knees is abnormal during movement and remains so. A less than perfect fit will lead to trouble even if the obesity does not last into adult life.

Children may become overweight for various reasons which are not well understood. They may eat a little too much or take too little exercise for a time so that the imbalance between input and output leaves behind a surplus of fat, or they may have laid down too many fat cells as babies. Mothers nowadays are severely discouraged from overfeeding their infants. Vicars and prospective MPs must understand that fat pink arms are not fashionable at baby shows any more; fat babies are not necessarily healthy babies after all.

Obesity is often a complication of other handicaps which have reduced the capacity for activity. A vicious circle is then set up in which the increasing weight produces a further reduction in activity levels. The sad truth is that having become fat it is hard to slim again whether you are a child or an adult. It is often forgotten that exercise can play a useful part along with controlled diet in getting rid of the extra weight. There will be more about this in Chapter 12.

The benefits of exercise must always be balanced against the risks. Strenuous physical activity in contact sports like rugby football is bound to produce frequent minor injuries but they soon heal. Keen team members always have a selection of cuts, scars, and bruises ready to display as evidence of their devotion. Major injuries involving broken bones are less frequent but sometimes cause permanent damage.

Competitive sport puts a premium on very high levels of performance from talented youngsters. There is a strong incentive to compete regardless of whether last week's injury is fully healed or next week's flu has just begun. This is a cause for concern because of the risk of permanent damage.

Overuse can cause damage even in an apparently innocent activity like running. Although there are no sudden stresses or violent collisions, running for long periods on hard surfaces can cause stress fractures, for instance at the top of the shin bone. This is a crack in the bone which causes pain and requires rest for healing but not complete immobilization. Gritting of the teeth and going on running will only make matters worse.

Similarly, excessive and prolonged stresses and strains on joints can cause damage to joint surfaces if they are vulnerable. Certainly during childhood and puberty persistent pain in a joint requires an adequate explanation before vigorous exertion is safe. The ends of certain bones sometimes become soft unexpectedly. This condition, known as osteochondritis, is unexplained and is probably not itself related to exercise. However, stresses and strains involved in rigorous exercise may be excessive for the bone in this state. They may lead to a permanent change in that part of the bone which forms the joint leaving a legacy of permanent damage and arthritis. Long bones grow by the progressive transformation of a plate of cartilage which separates the shaft of the bone from the end. This forms a joint with the next bone and is called an epiphysis. Growth finishes when the shaft and the epiphysis are finally joined by bone rather than cartilage. During growth there is always the possibility that the alignment between the shaft and the epiphysis will be upset by excessive loading. Therefore for young children and the gangly ill-coordinated adolescent long-distance running, high jumping, trampolining, and prolonged athletic contests are best attempted in small doses without too much competitive pressure.

There is no evidence that cardio-vascular damage occurs in normal healthy youngsters even in the most demanding sports such as cross-country skiing when the oxygen uptake and heart rate are at near maximum levels for quite long periods.

The sudden deaths which have occasionally been reported on the sports field have always been traced either to a pre-existing abnormality of the heart or circulation, or to a virus infection. Since virus infections can affect the heart, like rheumatic fever used to do, it is unwise for anyone to go out and play in a match if he or she has a raised temperature or feels unwell.

Sport is often considered a valuable outlet for aggression particularly in adolescent males. There is no evidence that aggression is reduced by competitive sport although various groups have examined the proposition. On the contrary, aggressive personality characteristics which were not previously apparent in youngsters are sometimes fostered by the adult aspirations surrounding team games and competitive sport. The archetypal school coach is a man who terrifies the weaklings, bullies the incompetent, swears at everyone, and enjoys enormous esteem because the team will win the Inter-Schools League. He is beloved of the favourites who aspire to the first team and heartily loathed by the rest who are also the many.

The aggressive energy of young children can be successfully channelled into physical activities which are creative and non-competitive. If these activities provide an opportunity for spontaneous self-expression and the release of feelings then the child can acquire more self-understanding and a better ability to communicate with others. Perhaps the disco has done more for our children than the decathlon.

The acquisition of motor skills is known to contribute towards meeting the basic psychological needs of safety and esteem in young children of both sexes and in adult adolescent boys. If we can do things effectively we feel better. The rub is that the motor skills demanded for school sports and physical education are high, and there is only room at the top for a few. The perpetual losers who have little natural aptitude are therefore the failures. Organized physical activity in school has for them resulted in increased feelings of inferiority and insecurity. Is it any wonder that so many adults react so badly when the word 'exercise' is mentioned?

Perhaps we should think very seriously about the objectives and consequences of games and physical education in school. What happens to the exuberant joy of the 7-year-old? Where has it gone when he is 17, 27, 57? Give a young child a wide open space, a field, or an empty gymnasium and he will run like the wind intoxicated by his own energy and the freedom to give it expression. This in some form should be part of our heritage when we are adults too.

4

WOMEN AND EXERCISE

The weaker sex?

Traditionally it has been men who have borne the brunt of heavy physical work and although it may be true that 'women's work is never done' their work has on the whole been lighter in kind. The extremist fringe of the women's liberation movement may feel indignant but there is sound biological justification for this. On average men are bigger than women, and they are also more muscular so that even when matched for size women have on average only 80 per cent of the strength of men. The men are therefore better equipped for physical work. However, it should not be forgotten that there is considerable overlap between the sexes in size and strength and there are plenty of women who are bigger and stronger than the average man. There are no less than 2,500 female miners in the United States. Also a man who sits at his desk all day and takes no exercise may have a lower exercise capacity than a woman who is looking after a house and young children.

The Olympics are still divided according to sex. However, in sports in which sheer body size is not an advantage the women can now achieve nearly as much as the men. Women have taken part in trans-Atlantic yacht races, swum the Channel, climbed Annapurna, and beaten male records for marathon hill-walking.

Women tend to have more body fat than men which accounts for their more curvaceous shape. And this is biologically determined by their genes. Because of their fat stores they will tolerate starvation for longer than men and because of their better insulation they will survive immersion in cold water for longer. These are dubious advantages since, when it comes to walking upstairs or climbing a hill, fat is a passenger and the muscles, whatever their size, have to perform more work. The second inevitable disadvantage is that haemoglobin levels in women tend to be lower than in men so the oxygen-carrying capacity of their blood is slightly less and this will reduce their performance capacity. If allowance is made for these two factors then women would be able to transport as much oxygen per kilogram of body weight as the men, provided that they were also prepared to train themselves as hard.

Almost the whole range of sport and exercise is open to women now, although preferences remain. Few women want to play football or practise weight-lifting although there is no reason why they should not.

All the rules of training which were explained in Chapter 2 apply to women as well as to men. Training is specific; leg work will not make arm work easier and vice versa. The overload principle applies; an increase in physical activity produces improvements and a decrease deterioration.

Exercise does not have a masculinizing effect on women. It takes years of weight-lifting to develop bulging muscles, and there are no significant changes in sex hormones. Rhythmic exercise is likely to improve a woman's appearance especially if it improves her posture. Well-trained muscles produce confident and graceful movement, and the spring in the step of a woman with energy to spare is attractive in itself.

There are large numbers of very inactive people of both sexes around today and many of the most inactive are women. They seem to have reduced their role in life to that of onlookers. Have they chosen this, or have they been edged out? It seems, from the outside, to be an undesirable disengagement from the enjoyable variety of human activity. If in young and middle-aged women the range of physical expectation is already so shrunken, what will old age hold in store?

An illusion which has been cherished by both men and women is that women and girls should be protected from physical activity in case they suffer harm, and more particularly in case their specifically female reproductive organs get damaged. The uterus (womb) is actually very securely anchored in the bony frame of the hips and will not shake loose or fall out! Provided there is no internal structural abnormality there is no reason why girls or women should not compete in the most strenuous sports including the long or high jump during any part of the menstrual cycle. This has been amply demonstrated by athletic women and some have carried off Olympic medals during their menstrual periods.

Fifty years ago exercise was considered dangerous for menstruating women especially if their periods were painful, then twenty years ago exercise was advocated as a cure for this common female misery. There is no evidence for either view and it appears now that exercise will do no harm but neither will it help. Since the pain is probably due to cramp-like spasm of the muscular walls of the uterus this is not surprising. This muscle, like any other, becomes painful if it is contracted in a sustained way for too long. The contraction blocks the blood flow, there is a local shortage of oxygen and a local build-up of metabolic end-products of energy release which cause the pain.

Claims have also been made for exercise as a palliative for premenstrual tension but again there is no good evidence. Active sportswomen are found to suffer less from premenstrual headaches than the inactive but this does not prove that the activity prevents the headaches.

There is only one group of women who are at greater risk from exercise than their male counterparts. As people grow older their bones become more brittle. Women, after the menopause, are worse off than men in this way and are more likely to suffer from broken bones.

Pregnancy is another time when women have sometimes been protected, perhaps too much, from physical activity. Certainly strenuous training before pregnancy does not have any adverse effects. Athletes are reported to have fewer miscarriages, a lower incidence of high blood pressure during pregnancy, and a shorter duration of the second stage of labour. These benefits may be due to good natural endowment rather than exercise but at least it is clear that the kind of strenuous training which produces a high physical working capacity and strong abdominal muscles does not have any adverse effects on subsequent pregnancy and may even be of benefit.

So much for exercise before the pregnancy begins. What about exercise other than relaxation classes during pregnancy? The instinctive response of many people to a full-bellied woman is to lead her gently by the hand to a chair. This may sometimes be appropriate in the last month or so of pregnancy. She will be grateful if she has spent the morning shopping and cleaning, but irritated if she was hoping for an invigorating walk. Exercise is of benefit to pregnant women and indeed important right up to the end of pregnancy and even into the first stage of labour provided they have adequate rest as well. In one study of a 26-week physical training programme for pregnant women considerable improvements in exercise tolerance were reported with no disturbance of the pregnancy and subsequent birth. Moreover, women who retain a good capacity for exercise until late in pregnancy have been found to have heavier babies. These women may belong to a selected group who have several natural advantages, so it would not be fair to claim that the babies are heavier because the mothers took plenty of exercise. Again the evidence is circumstantial. However, second and third babies are normally heavier than the first-born, which could be because of the greater physical demands made on a pregnant woman who already has several children. It is certainly true that during the last months of pregnancy the energy expenditure of a woman is bound to be high because of her extra weight, unless she stays in bed, and this is especially so if she already has other small children to look after.

For this reason alone it would seem sensible not to let exercise capacity dwindle during the earlier months. Circulatory capacity improves greatly early in pregnancy in anticipation of the increased demands which will be made by the growing foetus. There is no reason to allow the muscles to deteriorate, so that exercise becomes a drag. Women normally feel very well during the middle months of pregnancy and they should make the most of this.

In summary, leaving aside the rancour of chauvinist arguments from both male and female camps, the biological facts are first of all that women are on average a little smaller in size than men and tend to carry more fat, so their maximum strength and maximum capacity for high-intensity work is bound to be lower in general. However, this should not be used as an excuse for making little use of the considerable physical capacities which are there, because the second biological fact is that women respond to training and increased exercise in exactly the same way as men do, and their capacity for endurance exercise can be just as good as that of men. Although their sheer muscle strength is less their flexibility and stamina are just as good.

5

THE ELDERLY AND EXERCISE

Disuse or disease?

Comparisons between old and young are as fraught with rivalry as comparisons between men and women. On average, older people have a lower capacity for exercise than young people so it looks as though the passing years bring with them a slow loss of physical abilities. Muscle strength, flexibility, and stamina all tend to diminish with age. However, there are any number of exceptions and many 60-year-olds can do as much if not more than a 20-year-old of a similar size. Obviously the loss of physical capacities does not happen at the same rate for everyone, nor does it happen at a uniform rate for one person. There are many factors which affect capacity for exercise some of which are linked to age. There probably is some inevitable deterioration in body systems with the passage of time, in addition the accumulated effects of disease may produce a deterioration which appears to be age based, and finally dwindling physical activity levels in the elderly may well be a cause rather than a result of reduced physical capabilities.

The inevitable component of the deterioration in physical capacities with increasing age is due to irreversible biological changes: for example, the tissues become less elastic and resilient. The skin, for example, acquires bags and wrinkles. In the lungs the loss of elasticity means that less air will come out of the lungs at the end of each breath, and so the maximum ventilation rate is reduced. There is also a slow progressive loss of nerve cells which, unlike many other cells, cannot be replaced once they have died although the fibres in the nerve trunk can sometimes regrow if damaged. Little is known about the rate of cell loss but it will mean that some muscle cells are effectively lost, not because they are worn out but because their nerve supply has died. All these losses will reduce the maximum available muscle strength and maximum exercise capacity but will not necessarily impair the way in which the ageing body responds to moderate exercise demands.

Apart from the inevitable losses which may be slight in their effects, there are many chronic diseases which affect exercise capacity. These diseases may interfere directly with physical abilities or produce low levels of activity more indirectly because the disease causes a general malaise or a fear that exercise may exacerbate the condition. Some of these fears are groundless and this will be discussed in Part II. Since these diseases may take years to become manifest they affect the old more than the young. Two of the commonest of these conditions are arthritis and bronchitis. There are also cardio-vascular diseases like atherosclerosis which is the name given to the hardening and narrowing of the arterial blood-vessels. They become furred up like the plumbing in hard-water districts so that the blood supply to the heart muscle or the leg muscles may be severely reduced. All of these are common disabling conditions of the elderly for which there are palliatives but no real cures.

Apart from disease and age itself, a common disabling condition of the elderly is likely to be inactivity and for this there is a cure which is simple and costs no money. The effects of exercise or lack of it are not influenced by age. Inactivity will allow muscles to grow weaker, joints stiffer, and the cardio-vascular system less effective in elderly people just as much as in the young. Therefore much of the apparent loss of exercise capacity in elderly people is probably not a consequence of age at all but of lack of activity.

Once this was realized, exercise programmes and keep fit classes for the elderly began to be organized. Several studies of such programmes have been made, some using suitable control groups. The results show that the decline with age in endurance exercise capacity (stamina) is very much slower in groups who deliberately take some extra exercise.

One remarkable study in Russia supported claims that the normal decline can not only be slowed down but stopped completely or even reversed, so that there is no deterioration in physical working capacity with age at all. This study spanned ten years; at the beginning of it the age range of the participants was 51 to 74 years. The programme consisted of supervised group exercises twice a week for ninety minutes, similar daily exercises at home, and a variety of activities such as walking, skiing, or rambling. Maximum breathing capacity improved and resting blood pressure dropped a little. This indicates improvement in function of the respiratory and cardio-vascular systems. There were also improvements in the time taken to recover from exertion, improvements in balance, muscle strength (including arms, trunk, and leg muscles), and exercise performance measured in various ways (including running, jumping, and gymnastics). So the muscles were also capable of improvement and maintenance of capacity. There was no change in blood chemistry except for a rise in cholesterol during the last year. So there were improvements in almost all the measured abilities and functional attributes except the precision of hitting a target with a tennis ball! The improvements reached their peak after the first three to five years and were then maintained. By the end of the ten-year study the oldest participant was 81 years old. At a time when their contemporaries were declining in physical abilities this group either showed no deterioration or improved. It is obviously not practical to run exercise programmes on this scale for large numbers of the elderly but the message is clear. Each one of us as we grow older has a responsibility not to allow our bodies to let us down unnecessarily.

More evidence that the elderly can and do remain fit for demanding physical exercise comes from exceptional groups around the world and from exceptional individuals. There are communities in Vilcabamba in South America, Georgia in Southwest Russia, the Hunza and the Tarahumara tribes in Northern India in which the old continue to work and contribute physically to the life of their group. These are mainly agrarian societies in which levels of physical activity are high. The legendary ages of the old in these communities are still in dispute but undoubtedly they maintain a remarkably good exercise capacity despite their wrinkled skin and white hair. There is also a group in the United Kingdom in Norfolk living active lives in a country community until a ripe old age.

There are veteran cycling clubs whose members range up to 65 years of age, who still take part in 100-mile time-trials, clocking up scores only marginally below those of twenty or thirty years before. There are individuals who have begun jogging at the age of 60 and have gone on to run marathons. In the United Kingdom there is even a man aged 70 who climbs the rigging of the *Cutty Sark* every morning just for the hell of it, and intrepid elderly bathers who swim in the sea even in the winter. These things may not be for all of us but they show what can be done.

Society conspires, perhaps subconsciously, to keep the elderly in their armchairs and out of the action. 'Take it easy,' we say to our old folk, 'you have earned a rest.' We urge them to be cautious, not to overdo it. All in the name of promoting their health and prosperity into a ripe old age. We are probably doing them more harm than good. In keeping with social expectations, activity levels drift slowly and insidiously downwards with increasing age. The change is so slow that no one realizes that it is happening, or bothers to reverse it.

The influence of changes in physical activity levels on one's sense of well-being was by chance vividly illustrated when a group of factory workers in Poland gave up very heavy work. The incident occurred when a factory was closed down. The men who had been doing very strenuous work were moved to another factory and suddenly found themselves with jobs that were a good deal lighter than those to which they were accustomed. After a few weeks many of them went to see their doctors complaining that they felt vaguely unwell. They said that they were tired and that in particular they had no energy for digging their gardens at the week-ends. They were not ill. The reduction in exercise levels on the job was sufficient to lower their general fitness for work. They had noticed these effects only because the reduction in activity was so sudden. There are many good reasons why elderly people should not work as hard as Polish factory workers but the account of what happened to them underlines the reasons why the elderly as well as younger people should remain as active as possible.

Once he has become inactive an old person may find it harder than a young person to summon up the determination to increase activity levels again. There is little incentive from the outside to help motivate him, no demands to get back to work, so it is all too easy to slump. Minor illness or a bout of arthritis would leave all of us lacking in energy and easily tired but an elderly person often sees this as the final straw and decides to give up his allotment. This is quite unnecessary because once the cold or arthritic episode has cleared up, he can slowly regain the lost energy. If he does a little more each day he can return over a period of weeks to hoeing and weeding with the same enthusiasm as before. All but the most tenacious elderly people put their lack of energy after illness and inactivity down to old age and assume the dilapidation is permanent instead of temporary.

The effects of exercise and training on body systems are essentially the same at any age, and this has been demonstrated many times. Improvement will be easy for an inactive elderly person, not because of increased age but because he starts from a low level of activity. The principle of overload applies and so an extra walk every day, gradually increasing in speed and distance, will produce noticeable improvements within a few weeks. Just as with younger groups, the maximum capacity for exercise goes up and moderate exercise can be tolerated for longer without fatigue. Everyday tasks like cleaning the house will feel less tiring.

The physical capacity to go on living independently is of prime importance to the elderly and can only be preserved by taking a little more exercise rather than a little less. Energy resources will not be used up by the extra exercise, except in the very short term; it isn't as if one were born with a seventy-year supply. A good safety margin of physical capacity can be maintained by taking a little more than the bare minimum of exercise; minor set-backs due to illness are then less likely to be permanently disabling or to precipitate a final unwelcome admission to an old people's home or similar institution.

For younger people endurance exercise produces the most rewarding all-round improvements in exercise capacity. However, the proper maintenance of body systems, which will then equip their owner to face all the varied physical demands of daily life with equanimity, depends upon two more things as well as endurance capacity or stamina and these are joint flexibility and muscle strength. When activity levels and endurance capacity are very low, as they often are in the elderly, then the second two things need attention as well.

Joint flexibility may be at especial risk in the elderly because if arthritic pain leads to disuse of a joint for a time, it then seizes up. A full range of movement in all joints can be maintained or restored by gentle rhythmic movements regularly performed. This is especially important for the shoulder joint. The number of old ladies who have to ask a neighbour to do up the zip on the back of their dress might be fewer if more attention was paid to maintaining joint movement. The chiropodist is one of the most welcomed sources of paramedical help for the elderly not only to relieve the corns and bunions produced by seventy years of carrying 70 kilograms (154 pounds) about in ill-designed shoes, but also simply to cut toenails which can no longer be reached because their owner's spine and hips have become too stiff to allow him or her to bend down to touch them.

Lack of flexibility brings one set of problems, lack of muscle strength brings others. Getting up out of a low armchair, for instance, requires enough leg muscle to straighten the knee against the pull of gravity acting on most of the body mass (all of it except the feet and shins). This is a situation in which a combination of obesity and weak muscles spells disaster. A safety margin in muscle strength is a wise insurance not only for getting out of chairs but also against the damage which can occur if ligaments and tendons are submitted to sudden stresses. This can happen if one muscle gives way and suddenly all the others have to provide

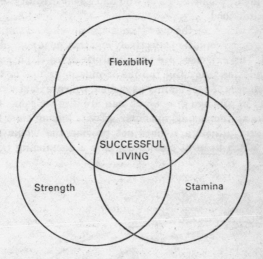

Fig. 6. The three requirements for successful living

extra support, due to an accidental push from a trolley in the supermarket, or an attempt to lift something too heavy. Muscle strength is developed and maintained by use, and so are flexibility and stamina, but it requires that the muscle is used at more than 80 per cent of its maximum strength for repeated short periods. This has been explained in Chapter 2. It means that the gentle exercise which maintains joint mobility and some endurance capacity may not be enough to maintain adequate muscle strength. Books describing exercises for the elderly are available now and many of the exercises which build up muscle strength can be performed unobtrusively at the bus stop, in a chair, or in bed. It is worth paying attention to the all-important trunk muscles because they support the spine which is central to all movements.

Swimming is a form of exercise which is valuable for developing all three aspects of good physical condition: flexibility, strength, and stamina. It is especially suitable for the elderly because the body's weight is largely supported by the water, and sudden movements are cushioned, so there are no undue stresses on joints which may be arthritic or bones which may be brittle. If the water is warm, tense muscles relax more easily. There are now swimming clubs run specially for the elderly to cater for those who are hesitant about public baths or who had no opportunity to learn to swim in childhood.

DANCE

Keep fit classes for the over-sixties also develop all three aspects of good physical condition effectively and they do it very pleasantly to music. The exercises are based on principles of physiotherapy and include the use of all the major muscle groups in the body. Keep fit classes appeal mainly to women, who are in any case more numerous in this age group, but men are also welcome. Old-time dancing is an increasingly popular activity among older men and women; and although it does not provide the whole range of exercise which keep fit classes do, it is a demanding endurance

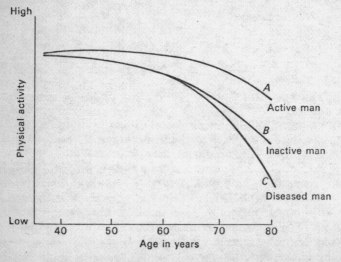

High

Physical activity

A
Active man

B
Inactive man

C
Diseased man

Low

40   50   60   70   80
Age in years

Fig. 7. The decline in physical activity with age

exercise which will also contribute something to joint flexibility and control of balance. Exercise should be a pleasure, not a burden, neither should it be taken like medicine. The elderly as well as the young should be able to find ways of keeping fit which are also fun.

We could probably all name at least one elderly person of our acquaintance who is outstandingly active and greatly enjoys life. Such people are remarkable because they are unusual. We do not say, 'Isn't he marvellous?' but, 'Isn't he marvellous for his age?' Are these people biologically special? They are physically robust having escaped debilitating diseases through luck, good management of their lives, or a genetically determined immunity. They are also psychologically robust enough to have rejected the normal life patterns of their peer group. We should look to them as appropriate examples of normal old age rather than to the more typical inactive 70-year-old. If the average values for physical ability in the population are lowered by disease, then they must not be accepted as norms to which the healthy should aspire. The 80-year-old who can still cover a good distance each day on foot or on his bicycle is normal, not peculiar, and the quality of his life in old age is unquestionably superior to that of other 80-year-olds who never go out of the house because they can only shuffle from bed to chair and back again.

6

PSYCHOLOGICAL EFFECTS OF EXERCISE

Feeling great?

Many benefits have been claimed for exercise over and above its improvement of muscles. Sometimes it is made to sound like a panacea for all ills, both physical and mental, a cure for almost anything except baldness. What can be said about the widely held views that exercise relieves insomnia, depression, minor mental illness, and general malaise; or about the idea that exercise can make you feel better even though you feel perfectly well in the first place?

'Feeling great!' was a slogan which was used by the Health Education Council of Great Britain and the British Broadcasting Corporation in a campaign in 1978 to encourage people to be more active. What lies behind this claim that exercise makes you feel great? It was certainly justified but on mainly rather prosaic grounds which must have been known by our ancient ancestors even though they did not understand the underlying reasons. We have recently come to understand the reasons a little better but there is no sensational new evidence to add to the old wisdom.

The first thing to be said is that there are psychological benefits which arise directly from improvements in muscle and exercise capacity. Over a longer time span there may be social consequences of improved exercise capacity which lead to psychological benefits for social reasons, an indirect effect of increased exercise. These two things may improve life for anyone. Thirdly, there is now reliable evidence that exercise can help in some forms of minor mental illness.

After a programme of exercise training many groups report that they feel better either spontaneously or in response to a questionnaire. It is hard to know whether this rather general feeling is the result, either directly or indirectly, of physical improvements, whether it is due to a more specific effect of exercise on states of mind, or whether it is just a consequence of the care and attention received from those running the exercise programme. Some attempts have been made to sort out these various possibilities.

Direct effects are obviously the easiest to investigate and among the long-term benefits one which has been thoroughly studied recently is the change in perception of effort. After training, physical work feels easier, the perception of effort is less, and this can be explained by physical factors. The increase in the strength of muscles and of their capacity to take up and use oxygen to do work means that any given task is now less of an effort. The task taxes a smaller fraction of the muscles' maximum ability and so feels easier. For people to be able to face the physical demands of daily living knowing that they will feel less of a burden undoubtedly improves the quality of life. There is energy to spare which can restore a bounce to the step and reawaken a zest for living. This can be counted a psychological benefit.

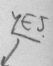

Of even greater interest and importance to mental health are the secondary changes which may follow these physical changes. If work feels easier, this may bring relief from anxiety about physical abilities and a greater physical delight in bodily movement.

Moreover, if physical capacities improve, more involvement in active social pursuits becomes possible, and this in turn may lead to a richer variety of social relationships. This is particularly important for the elderly. If it is too tiring to walk down the road to watch a bowls match or collect the evening paper, then a keenly debated discussion about the youngest player's form and some local gossip from the corner shop are lost as well. Friendships as well as muscles dwindle from lack of use. Life takes a downward turn in a vicious self-propagating spiral leading away from physical activity and the social involvement which it allows. This may seem a drastic example but even in younger age groups, joining the squash club or the rambling association can change a restricted and therefore lonely life into a full and happy one. The scales can be tipped in this way by involvement in social clubs of many sorts which do not necessarily involve physical activity, but having some spare physical capacity keeps more options open.

This may be the explanation for the claim that exercise improves sexual activity. Making love can be physically demanding and so a good exercise capacity is useful, but more than that, feelings of physical well-being and a positive attitude to life are likely to enhance sexual experience or diminish it if they are absent. The old theory, rife in boys' public schools, that exercise provides an alternative outlet for sexual drive has no justification except in the very short term. After strenuous activity people want rest, not more activity of any kind, but this soon wears off.

In addition to the psychological consequences of physical improvements, whether they are direct or indirect, exercise may have specific effects on the behaviour, personality, and states of mind of normal people. These things are difficult to measure and it is difficult to disentangle the social effects of an exercise programme from the effects of the exercise itself. However, there are a few controlled studies which suggest that there are specific psychological effects. Normal adults become more extrovert, more self-confident, more understanding, and more self-aware after exercise programmes. Obviously only those who initially lack these attributes will show changes. One might debate whether increased extroversion is beneficial but there is evidence that extroverts cope better with disruptions like moving house or a trauma like bereavement. Self-confidence, understanding, and self-awareness are surely to be desired without reservation. These changes are small in degree and seem likely to outlast the original exercise programme better than the changes in muscle function, but there is no evidence that this is so. It could be claimed that exercise produces personality changes which sounds a little threatening, but it seems much more likely that what the exercise is doing is to restore lost self-confidence and self-awareness or to allow the realization of potential capacities for understanding or extroversion.

A commonly believed but unsubstantiated piece of exercise lore is that exercise provides an outlet for aggression. It is possible that aggressive energies can be channelled into socially acceptable physical contests either against opponents, a ball, or one's own record. Many people say they find it helpful to unleash pent-up frustrations by hitting a ball as hard as possible. This may be a form of catharsis. On the other hand there is no evidence that sport reduces aggressive behaviour in youngsters. Those who have looked for such evidence have found the reverse. There is also evidence that competitive sport, organized by adults for children, fosters competitive assertive attitudes in the children. It looks as though the competitive tendencies inherent in a capitalist society are being foisted on to the children through the medium of sporting activities, all in the name of providing them with an outlet for their 'aggression'.

Success in sport brings increased self-confidence to children, but for every success there are failures which bring frustration and crushed self-esteem. A new kind of tug-of-war game has been suggested, a much more challenging game than the old one. The object of the new game is not to pull the other team over the line but to keep the rope in play, so if you detect an imminent win for your side, you let go and rush round to help the other team.

A good capacity for exercise should still be thought of as a necessary tool for satisfactory living, necessary for full mental health as well as physical well-being.

Motivation for maintaining exercise capacity varies as much as the recipe for achieving it. Some people find exercise a delightful end in itself. They have rediscovered the physical pleasures of using well-trained muscles and find that running or swimming makes them feel good at the time as well as later. Some people even describe feelings of euphoria and elation during vigorous exercise. This may explain why some people get addicted to exercise; it becomes a compulsive activity and they say they feel irritable if they are deprived of it.

However, not all of us find pleasure in jogging. For some the only pleasure is the relief when it stops. This is not entirely due to an inadequate physical capacity which would improve with practice. There are also sportsmen with plenty of athletic ability who enjoy their sport but do not get a euphoric kick out of running for its own sake. This is a good example of the way in which physical ability is a tool which allows the enjoyment of a chosen sport.

But what are the alternatives for those who do not like running or cycling and have no interest in sport? Some have recently responded to campaigns to jolt them into activity by taking exercise like medicine three times a week. If they are motivated by fear of heart attacks or other illnesses then this seems a particularly unfortunate outcome. Groups of jogging hypochondriacs are not what the exercise campaign organizers intended to create. In any case a personal exercise programme pursued out of fear is not likely to last long. We need to build some physical activity into our daily lives on a permanent basis and in a way which is not dreary. Substituting a walk to work instead of a bus or car journey might mean the beginning of an enjoyable routine, or better still acquire a dog who will insist on his rights, which consist of two walks a day whatever the weather. Exercise does not have to be a punishment; if it is felt as such it is not likely to bring psychological benefits.

So far the effects of exercise on normal mental health have been considered, what about its effects on impaired mental health?

Carefully controlled studies have shown that people with behavioural and emotional difficulties can, through exercise, improve in self-acceptance and develop more positive emotional and intellectual behaviour. There seem to be parallels here with the mental changes brought about in normal individuals by exercise. Self-awareness and self-confidence may have common ground with self-acceptance and positive emotional behaviour. The labels change according to the many different psychological tests used, but the same general message emerges. Exercise does have welcome effects on mental function.

Exercise has also been suggested as a cure for minor mental illnesses and depression. This may be too big a claim. There is no sound evidence for substantiating or rejecting it. However, since psychological benefits are much more difficult to measure than physical ones it seems wise to give exercise the benefit of the doubt. It will certainly have fewer unpleasant side-effects than sleeping tablets and tranquillizers. These are doled out nowadays in large quantities and at great expense. In a recent survey, 15 per cent of car drivers were found to be under the influence of drugs other than alcohol. Exercise is worth a serious try. It might even be possible that lack of exercise has contributed to the development of minor degrees of mental illness and that if the drivers could be got out of their cars and set on their feet they could cure themselves.

Chronic insomnia is another common manifestation of imperfect mental health but controlled studies have failed to show that exercise helps people to sleep better. Again lack of evidence does not prove that exercise has no effect on sleep, merely that if there is an effect it is too small to show, or that it only works for a few people. If the effect is too small to show then it is not of much use, but if it works for some people clearly it may be of great use to them. This variation in the way different people respond bedevils research and leaves plenty of room for speculation and assertions based on one or two selected cases, which then become accepted dogma. As with mental illness and exercise, we do not know the answers and so if you are an insomniac it would be worth trying a late-night workout instead of counting sheep.

Sleep problems are usually trivial compared with the problems facing mentally handicapped children. Such children probably need deliberately fostered play activity in order to develop as fully as possible both physically and mentally. Studies have shown that educationally subnormal boys and mentally retarded children improved in mental tests after an exercise programme. The improvements may have been due to a change in attitude or the positive emotional effects of physical achievement. Moreover, achievement of any kind might have produced similar results but, whatever the mechanism and whether or not it is specific to exercise, the benefits are real, valuable, and not difficult to bring about. Other studies have shown that children with mental handicaps resulting in severe lack of muscular co-ordination can also, perhaps surprisingly, benefit from exercise programmes. This is because they gain in self-confidence and self-esteem.

At the other end of the age spectrum, geriatric mental patients were also found to benefit from exercise. This is a group with multiple problems. They tend to be written off as being beyond hope or help except by a dedicated handful of the medical profession and yet, for them too, exercise produces improvements. Several controlled studies have shown that an exercise programme is feasible even with such a difficult group and that it can produce improved mental function, better short-term memory, and more acceptable social behaviour. Again, whatever the underlying mechanism the changes are too valuable to be ignored.

Even if it doesn't make all of us feel great there is enough evidence to claim that exercise can bring mental as well as physical benefits. The Romans had words for it. It was Juvenal who said 'Mens sana, in corpore sano'. If exercise is neglected in a machine-powered age, life goes on but a whole dimension of refreshing variety has been lost. Machines will not usher in a new super race, we can be grateful to them according to their due but then turn back to re-evaluate the ancient wisdom. The capacity for physical exercise is a fundamental tool for successful living.

7

HAZARDS OF EXERCISE

The man who does nothing loses for certain

There are risks attached to any activity but perhaps the greatest risk in an exercise programme is that people will embark upon it too enthusiastically, misjudge their capacity, and make themselves so stiff and sore that they give up any further attempt to become fitter. They may also lose their resolve to take more exercise if their doctor, their family, or their favourite newspaper columnist is discouraging. So much effort has gone into removing physical activity from our lives that there is some reluctance to reverse the previous trend. The scientific and medical case for exercise has only been assembled in the last few years and we have mentioned in other chapters persisting uncertainties. Fatalities which may or may not be attributable to exercise programmes make headline news; the attempt to change attitudes is looked at suspiciously.

There are some hazards. They are greatly diminished by understanding and by respect for advice. Sudden excessive loads may damage bones, joints, ligaments, tendons, or muscles and occasionally in certain vulnerable individuals severe exercise may provoke potentially fatal disturbances of the heart's function.

Normally exercise generates stresses and strains which remain well within the tolerance limits of the body. Breathlessness and aching muscles bring us to a halt long before we get anywhere near the dangerous limits of self-destruction. However, rapid and powerful movements which do not in themselves cause damage can set up high accelerations which are dangerous if the movements are not well controlled or if accidents occur. Contact sports such as rugby, soccer, and also skiing are the activities most likely to cause damage. Running down a steep slope is, surprisingly, more hazardous than running uphill. Muscles are most vulnerable to injury when they fail to contract smoothly. When running downhill, the muscles have to lengthen and, as it were, let the body weight fall in a controlled manner. This represents a great strain and the muscles may lengthen jerkily. Weary muscles and cold muscles may also fail to contract smoothly. Hence the need for gradual warming up before strenuous exercise.

The risks are greater without preliminary training because the muscles and tendons are weak. Moreover, those who are over-weight because they are fat rather than because they have large muscles are at greater risk than the small and thin, because their momentum is increased without a matching increase in muscular power. Their strength to weight ratio is low like an underpowered car which has poor brakes and is laden with too many passengers. Among these people are the dads who go out to play football with energetic sons and find themselves in pain for months with strains and sprains or worse.

The young bounce better than the middle-aged for a number of reasons. Their muscles and tendons are made of basically similar material but their body weight is much less so they develop less momentum in vigorous games and the effects of gravity are less. In addition, young tendons and bones are more resilient, less brittle than old ones, and young muscles are normally accustomed to exercise and therefore stronger for their size.

Even a stately jogging programme free from the rough and tumble of the scrum can produce minor sprains of joints and tendons. Minor problems can take a long time to clear up in middle-aged and elderly people so it is wise to get fitter by taking part in a wide variety of different physical activities which do not strain the same minor weaknesses. Overuse injuries range from inflamed tendons to stress fractures of the bones of the legs (cracks in the bone appearing with excessive use). If it hurts then rest it; discretion is the better part of valour. Then when it feels better gradually resume activity.

Jogging on roads presents certain hazards. If sore feet are to be avoided when running or walking any distance on hard surfaces well-padded shoes are needed. The risk of road traffic accidents is real and may often occur if fatigue is allowed to progress to the point where it impairs alertness. Special care should be taken when running near or on public highways, particularly at night. White or light-coloured clothes greatly improve the chance of being seen by motorists.

The second kind of hazard, that of overloading the cardio-vascular system, is quite different. Disasters are much rarer but much more serious if they occur. This is why they have had an undue amount of publicity, and set many faces against exercise quite unnecessarily. The heart does not get tired like skeletal muscles but various different kinds of cardio-vascular accidents can occur and almost all depend upon there being a weakness already present in the system. Sudden death on the sports field in those who are apparently young and healthy is always found to be due to some pathological cause which was already there.

Jogging has often been blamed by the press for unexpected deaths in middle-aged people. Many times a proper investigation of the story reveals that the exercise taken was blamed unjustly. On the other hand, many men and women are at risk from sudden exertion because they already have some degree of arteriosclerotic disease which affects the blood-vessels supplying the heart (see Chapter 8). These changes begin in adolescence and progress slowly unknown to their victims. This situation, coupled with a low level of physical fitness for exercise, leaves such people vulnerable to heart attack. Unaccustomed heavy exertion is unwise and the advice to get fitter by progressive modest increases in exercise is specially intended to get people better prepared for sudden exertion.

It used to be a common belief that missed heart beats, particularly when they occurred during exercise, were a sign that exercise was likely to cause sudden death. It is now known that over a third of normal people have missed beats on exercise, the incidence increasing with age. The evidence is that there is no reason why people with missed beats should restrict their exercise.

Those who already have heart disease may suffer pain across the chest, called angina, during exercise. This is due to the heart muscle having to work with an inadequate oxygen supply because the coronary blood-vessels are narrowed or blocked. The condition limits exercise. It is necessary to take medical advice the first time it occurs. Some investigation may prove necessary but it is usually possible to resume exercise, indeed it is desirable for the reasons already given. A little extra caution may be needed. A heart with a reduced coronary blood supply is vulnerable and sudden demands for a greatly increased work output from the heart may precipitate a disturbance of rhythm which could be fatal or cause irreversible damage to a part of the heart muscle.

Many diseases of the heart cause heart failure. This often makes ankles swell and limits exercise, severe breathlessness being caused by the slightest physical effort. The heart muscle is weakened by these diseases and cannot generate a sufficiently powerful contraction to pump effectively. However, modern treatment can often dramatically improve a patient's capacity for exercise and may well allow him to take regular walks. The heart does not fail from age alone so that the elderly are not at risk from their age in itself.

A small number of older people have a weakness of the wall of an artery (or aneurysm). Exercise is one of the many daily activities which can increase blood pressure. Any such rise, particularly in someone whose blood pressure is already raised, may lead to rupture of the aneurysm and bleeding into the surrounding tissue. If this happens in the brain it may cause brain damage known as stroke (see Chapter 8). The risk associated with exercise does not appear to be unduly great but it is the reason for advising individuals who already have high blood pressure to avoid sustained muscular effort of more than a few seconds' duration because of the large increases in blood pressure which it produces.

Fainting, during or after exercise, is alarming but it does not necessarily mean that the victim has had a heart attack. There will still be a pulse but it may be temporarily weak and difficult to detect. (Try the carotid pulse in the neck or the femoral in the groin if the radial pulse at the wrist is undetectable.) Fainting is due to loss of consciousness because the blood supply to the brain is inadequate. The horizontal posture is normally enough to restore the status quo within a minute. On no account should fainting persons be propped up. Fainting during exercise is very rare and much more serious than fainting afterwards. During exercise cardiac output, blood pressure, and blood flow to the brain all rise considerably unless the heart is failing to pump. This can happen because of a disturbance of rhythm or because the heart becomes embarrassed by the increased volume of blood it is required to pump (true heart failure). Fainting after exercise is not uncommon even in well-trained athletes if it has been heavy and particularly if the environment is hot. It occurs because the arteries of the exercising muscles and also those of the skin are widely dilated. The circulation requires the pumping action of the muscles to return venous blood to the heart so that it can maintain a sufficiently high output of blood to fill these dilated arteries and maintain the pressure. This is the reason for finishing a bout of exercise by continuing to exercise gently, thereby keeping the pumping action of the muscles going, rather than stopping abruptly and standing still.

Extremes of weather present hazards. Slippery road surfaces cause accidents but there are also more subtle threats. There have been accounts of death due to heart attack during snow-shovelling in middle-aged men in North America. These tragedies may be due simply to the unaccustomed exercise but they may have been exacerbated by a reflex spasm of coronary arteries due to the cold.

Hot weather also places an increased load upon the circulation. The dilatation of the skin arteries and the need for an increased blood flow through them is in itself an increased strain on the system. If there is also copious sweating the body may lose sufficient water and salts to reduce the blood volume which will embarrass the circulation further. Exercise programmes are better abandoned or postponed in very hot or very cold weather.

Exercise is better avoided after a heavy meal for similar reasons. The digestive system requires a large blood flow to maintain the flow of digestive juices and absorb the digested food. The circulatory system will therefore be embarrassed if exercise demands are added to the situation. There will be no failure of cardiac output in a healthy person but neither the digestion or the muscles will be adequately served because they are competing for the same supply. Indigestion, poor exercise performance, and cramp may result. Man is designed to eat or to work but not to do both to excess simultaneously.

Exercise should also be avoided during feverish illnesses because there is a chance of viral infection of the heart muscle of which the patient will be unaware. Strenuous exercise can damage the heart in such conditions. Rheumatic fever was a common disease of this kind years ago. During an attack of asthma, exercise is unwise, but between attacks exercise is often beneficial.

The risks involved in taking exercise are small provided common sense is used. Minor orthopaedic injuries are the most likely, especially in exuberant enthusiasts. These can be avoided by the sober middle-aged with proper caution. It cannot be said too often that cardio-vascular accidents caused by sensible exercise are very rare.

Both kinds of accident are less likely in those who are used to exercise. A deliberate campaign to increase activity levels gradually and safely will therefore reduce the risk of accidents caused by the sudden unexpected exercise demands of daily life. That run for the bus in order to keep a worrying appointment is less likely to end in disaster if running is nothing unusual. We cannot do better than borrow the British Safety Council's Sportsman's Safety Code:

1. The benefits of exercise come from a regular graduated programme. Decide which sport or activity you would like to adopt
   and establish that it is possible, in practical terms, for you to
   maintain regular participation.
2. There is nothing to be gained from over-exertion. A gentle
   progression to extend your limits is the best way.
3. The body needs time to regain agility and suppleness – unfamiliar movements are likely to cause sprains and strains.
4. The warm-up period before any sport is vital. Top professionals
   would not neglect it. A few simple stretching and loosening
   exercises even before jogging are essential.
5. Unused muscles are bound to ache but acute pain could be a
   warning sign of a heart attack or serious injury and should not
   be ignored.
6. Wear suitable clothes and the right protective equipment where
   required – with particular attention to footwear.
7. Do not undertake the 'hazardous' sports (climbing, canoeing,
   pot-holing) except under expert guidance and tuition.
8. All sports equipment should be of the highest possible quality,
   be well maintained, and be checked regularly.
9. As far as possible, participate in your sport with others, joining
   clubs or associations or forming small groups (e.g. jogging
   party). This will give you access to expertise, provide encouragement for flagging enthusiasm, and create an automatic supervi-
   sion.

Part II

EXERCISE AND DISEASE

This section is about people with known chronic diseases like asthma, disorders like obesity, and handicaps like arthritis. The instinct to protect these people from physical demands is not always appropriate because even more than healthy people they need to make the most of the physical potential which remains to them. Training effects are available to any individual who can manage regular exertion of some kind. There are no appreciable dangers provided common sense and a gradual approach are used. Any gain in effort tolerance and in work capacity for the tasks of daily life is worth a great deal to the disabled and may have a significant effect upon their capacity for independent living.

8

EXERCISE AND CARDIO-VASCULAR DISORDERS

Whodunnit?

The commonest cardio-vascular disorder is coronary heart disease (CHD) and a recent progressive increase in its prevalence among middle-aged men has been labelled an epidemic. A more sober assessment of the situation, which takes into account changes in the diagnoses favoured by doctors when completing death certificates, is less alarming. It suggests that its incidence has almost doubled in the last twenty years in males aged between 40 and 60 years. This is worrying but hardly qualifies as an epidemic. It can be explained in part, but only in part, by the change in the death rate from diseases like bacterial pneumonia and septicaemia which are now effectively controlled by antibiotics. So the hunt is on to try and find out what has contributed to the increase in the incidence of CHD and by implication how to stem it. First of all, what is coronary heart disease?

The usual cause of CHD is atherosclerosis of the coronary arteries. The inner layer of the arterial wall, which should be very smooth, becomes roughened. Fat and cholesterol are deposited in these roughened areas and the artery eventually blocks up, due to the deposits or because of a clot or thrombosis caused by the rough surface. The first changes are to be found in early adult life, even in childhood, and may develop on the basis of a congenital weakness of certain areas of the arterial wall. In many men, by middle age, the process has advanced to the stage when there may be a sudden obstruction of one of the three main coronary arteries with consequent death of a portion of the heart muscle supplied by that artery, a coronary thrombosis. Alternatively, as a result of the gradual narrowing of all three arteries there is a restriction of the blood supply to the heart and the needs of the heart for oxygen cannot be met under all conditions; consequently chest pain develops during exercise (angina). As the disease progresses the risk of a sudden change in the heart rhythm increases. The change in rhythm may have such an unfortunate effect on the heart's function that it can no longer work as a pump and sudden death occurs. This can happen before either a coronary thrombosis or angina have developed. However, many patients make a good recovery from a coronary thrombosis and both they and patients with angina may survive for many years.

There has been a hope recently that some of the changes involved in the development of CHD may be influenced for the good by regular exercise. Two questions come to mind. Does exercise slow down the progress of the disease? Could it ever cure it? The

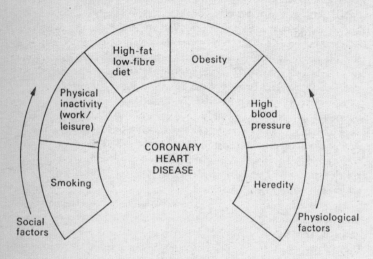

Fig. 8. Factors which may accelerate the progress of coronary heart disease

case is difficult to prove, since it takes thirty or forty years for the disease to become manifest. Controlled studies of the effects of activity are not possible and so the next best thing is to compare groups who are known to differ in activity levels.

The incidence of CHD is sometimes found to be less in groups of men who have physically active occupations or particularly active leisure pursuits. Studies of London busmen more than twenty years ago produced the first suggestion that physical activity was associated with a low risk of CHD. This study is difficult to interpret because the more sedentary drivers were also fatter, and obesity on its own can contribute to the development of CHD.

The most dramatic demonstration has been seen in the study of San Francisco's longshoremen (dockers) who were followed for twenty-two years (or to death or to age 75 years). Those men who were in very energetic jobs requiring repeated bursts of very hard work had a death rate from CHD almost half that found in men performing work which required a medium or low level of exertion. It should be realized that the level of work of most of the longshoremen was very high compared to that of the general population. This may therefore not lead to any very practical advice for the man in the street.

Those in sedentary jobs may have active leisure pursuits. A ten-year study of middle-aged sedentary male civil servants carried out in Britain has shown that those reporting vigorous exercise during leisure time had a lower incidence of CHD. It was one-third as prevalent as in a matched inactive control group. In this study vigorous exercise included contrived exercise and sport as well as heavy work in the garden, house, or garage. This is encouraging but studies of athletes have failed to show that they have an increased longevity or a reduction in the incidence of CHD which would be expected if exercise had a protective function.

If exercise does have an influence on the development of CHD, then what is the mechanism? There is no good evidence that the unwelcome changes in the arterial walls can be reversed by exercise, but their progress might be slowed down.

It was suspected for a long time that blood fats like cholesterol played a role in the development of atherosclerosis since the arterial thickening is largely due to fatty deposits. Sure enough, a high incidence of CHD was found to be associated with high cholesterol levels in blood. Of all the various risk factors this is the best predictor of CHD. However, that does not mean that it is a good predictor, only about 30 per cent of those suffering from CHD have high cholesterol levels, so what about the others? Moreover, exercise does not reduce the levels of cholesterol although it does reduce levels of other blood fats if they are abnormally high. So the story is confused. However, recently it has been observed that well-trained middle-aged men have higher levels of certain blood proteins than those who are sedentary. These are so-called high-density lipoproteins (HDLs) which bind cholesterol and by the part they play in transporting fat and cholesterol out of the blood-vessel wall reduce its possible damaging effects. This finding may be of particular significance since in a large group of Norwegian men the elevated blood levels of high-density lipoproteins have been shown to be related to a reduced prevalence of CHD, low levels being predictive of rapidly advancing disease. It may also explain the success with which the Masai people of Tanzania can tolerate a high-fat diet without succumbing to CHD. These people are nomadic and physically active sometimes walking about 110 kilometres (70 miles) in a day with their herds.

One of the immediate causes of death from CHD is the formation of a clot in a narrowed coronary artery, a coronary thrombosis. Does exercise have any effect on the likelihood of this happening? It is possible that exercise produces changes in the blood which make it less likely to clot. This could happen in three ways, through changes in the number or behaviour of platelets (small fragments of cells which initiate the coagulation of blood), through changes in the concentration or potency of a large number of clotting factors, or through changes in processes which dissolve blood clots once formed.

Short bouts of exercise certainly affect the levels of these substances, but the changes increase the tendency to clot. On the other hand, there is an increase in the power of the systems which can dissolve clots which compensates for the increased clotting tendency. In the short term no clear gain is evident. However, a small number of studies have compared the trained athlete with the sedentary individual and the results of such studies suggest a difference and indicate that training may reduce the possibility of blood clots forming at a site of damage to the blood-vessel wall and persisting there.

So far the possibility is still open that continued strenuous exercise slows down the development of CHD by altering the way in which cholesterol is carried in the blood and that exercise might reduce the tendency of the blood to clot once CHD is well advanced.

The next question is whether people who are used to exercise can survive and recover from a heart attack due to CHD better than those who are inactive. It has been suggested that exercise might improve the blood supply to the heart muscle in three possible ways. It might cause a widening of the main coronary arteries, or lead to the development of more medium-sized blood-vessels (collaterals) or a more prolific capillary network. There is no evidence for any of this although it must also remain a possibility.

The last suggestion followed the discovery that the capillary bed in muscles of the skeleton develops with exercise. The first from the story of a man called Clarence de Mar, who ran marathon races in the United States until he was in his sixties, and had very wide coronary arteries. Neither suggestion has been substantiated by research. An autopsy study in Britain did not reveal any convincing evidence for enlarged coronary arteries in men having a history of heavy occupational exertion. Those whose coronary arteries have become so narrow that the heart is seriously short of oxygen can be helped by coronary bypass surgery. A vein, perhaps from the patient's leg, where it is not indispensable, is used as a graft in place of the narrowed artery.

The pain caused by heart muscle working without an adequate oxygen supply (angina) has been mentioned in the last chapter. Training almost always ameliorates this condition, not because of improvements in the heart but because of the improvements in the muscles of the skeleton (normally leg muscles) which allow much more work to be done before anginal pain becomes limiting. In addition, after training heart patients can work at a given intensity with a lower cardiac output and a lower blood pressure. So the heart is spared in several ways by the improvements produced by exercise in working muscles and the circulation.

One of the most important effects of training for patients with angina or for those who are recovering from a heart attack is a psychological one. The gains in confidence which come from increasing exercise levels in a safely controlled way are as valuable as the physical gain. Instead of becoming 'cardiac cripples' many of these patients return to active lives and some have even gone on to participate in marathon running, a feat which was probably beyond their wildest dreams *before* they had the heart attack, let alone afterwards.

The heart is not the only organ which suffers from the damaging effects of atherosclerosis. The blood-vessels of the leg muscles can become blocked up in the same way resulting in pain on walking because the muscles are inadequately supplied with oxygen. Exercise can improve this condition by its effects on the capacity of the muscle cells to take up and use oxygen, and possibly also by promoting the growth of collateral bypass vessels. The evidence for the second effect is controversial since development of collaterals sometimes occurs anyway without much exercise.

When the blood-vessels of the brain are diseased this can sometimes result in the worst of all the cardio-vascular diseases which is a stroke. Areas of brain tissue die because of a disrupted blood supply. The resulting damage to the central nervous system is variable and often very debilitating. There is no evidence that exercise has any good effect but the search has not been as intensive as for CHD.

High blood pressure is another common and damaging cardio-vascular disorder in Western society. Exercise raises arterial blood pressure while it is in progress but conversely it has been shown that resting blood pressure comes down a little after training. The effect may be sufficient to allow the mild hypertensive to avoid drug therapy. This would be an important benefit but there have not yet been enough adequate long-term studies to establish this.

This inconclusive state of knowledge is not unusual where chronic diseases are concerned. If they take many years to develop and have multiple causes, then it is virtually impossible to do the controlled studies which are needed to unravel the story with certainty. Exercise helps by improving general muscle function and so reducing the strain of exercise on the circulation. Whether it also does more than that remains to be seen.

9

EXERCISE AND RESPIRATORY DISEASES

The English disease

In Britain, fog, air pollution, and cigarettes combine to produce more respiratory disease than anywhere else in the world. People with such diseases form the one group for whom inadequacy of the lungs limits exercise and it might seem that they would be the last group to benefit from it. However, the general rules hold good. Because exercise improves the muscles, it does improve the exercise tolerance of those with respiratory disease just as it does for anyone else, and increased confidence is an added bonus for those with chronic disease of this kind.

In chronic bronchitis the airways of the lung become narrowed by mucous cells and thick layers of mucus as well as by spasm of the muscle layer encircling the air passages so that the resistance to airflow is high and breathing becomes hard work. Eventually the disease progresses to a final stage when the patient can no longer breathe in enough air to keep his tissues adequately supplied with oxygen. Before that stage is reached there are many years of reasonably normal life interspersed with acute bouts of infection. Between such bouts bronchitics should not avoid exercise. They can train themselves without harm despite their breathlessness. Studies have shown that brisk walking and stair-climbing are effective in producing noticeable improvements in performance and exercise tolerance.

Emphysema is another degenerative disease fairly common in the elderly in which lung tissue loses its elasticity and air tends to be trapped in the lungs. This effectively reduces breathing capacity but these people also can achieve some improvement in their physical capacities safely with sensibly graded activity. Exercise will not cure bronchitis or emphysema but will enable the victims to live with it more comfortably. People with chronic respiratory disease should not relegate themselves prematurely to wheelchairs.

Asthma is a common respiratory disease which is something of a paradox because it is sometimes caused and sometimes helped by exercise. The symptoms are due to a narrowing of the airways just as in bronchitis. This is due to contraction of the muscle coats forming the walls of the airways. The degree of contraction varies from time to time. In some asthmatics the muscle coat is supersensitive and contracts in response to many things including inhaled foreign proteins. This is why cats, dogs, and feather beds can precipitate attacks of wheezing; asthmatics are allergic to small air-borne particles of protein from the fur. Endurance exercise can also trigger mild attacks of wheezing even in individuals who have not previously experienced the symptom. This is because of supersensitivity to cold dry air rather than the exercise itself. These individuals usually have close relatives with asthma, hay fever, or allergy. The problem may need treatment but can usually be controlled by a medicament spray used before exercise.

Asthmatics tolerate swimming and sprinting better than long-distance running, and many benefit from the usual muscular improvement produced by endurance exercise. More surprisingly, in several studies of the possible benefits of exercise in children, some lost their asthmatic symptoms partially or completely by persevering with exercise, although it induced symptoms at first. It is known that asthma may involve psychological factors and this may be why it is sometimes amenable to such dramatic improvement. It should also be remembered that some children grow out of asthma as they become adults.

Exercise between acute attacks of asthma is recommended, especially for children, even if it has to be achieved with the help of broncho-dilator drugs. The frequency of attacks of asthma decreases, and the intensity of exercise at which exercise-induced asthma occurs is much higher due to the general improvement of physical condition. Life is less restricted and there is less absence from school or work.

For many people with chronic respiratory disease exercise will not cause harm if it is sensibly organized and it can improve the quality of an inevitably restricted life, although it will not cure the disease or prolong life.

10

EXERCISE AND MUSCULO-SKELETAL DISORDERS

'A jog a day keeps the osteopath away'
(General Council and Register of Osteopaths)

There is still debate about the role of exercise in the development of the commonest musculo-skeletal disorder which is osteo-arthritis. Not everyone would agree with the osteopaths although there are good reasons for their views. Suitable exercise keeps joints lubricated and also maintains muscle strength, both of which in different ways protect joints from damage. Others believe that a lifetime of physical exercise can lead to degeneration of the joint surfaces due to overuse. These opposing views will probably be reconciled by defining exactly what is meant by physical exercise. The concept that materials 'fatigue' is not new following the publicity given to the occurrence of 'fatigue fractures' in aircraft such as the DC10's or Tridents.

It must be admitted that the cartilage of which joint surfaces are made is fatigue prone and therefore liable to mechanical failure. An important factor is the ability of the bone underlying the cartilage to act as a shock absorber. Continual sudden pressure, such as would be produced in the knees by jumping, may lead to stiffening of the bone in response to the loading. Bone is not a fixed tissue for all its solidity, it is constantly remodelling itself and it responds to increased stresses by thickening and stiffening. If the bone under the cartilage becomes stiffer then it is less effective as a shock absorber and so the cartilage is more vulnerable. Footballers, parachutists, pneumatic drillers, and the obese would therefore be expected to have a higher incidence of osteo-arthritis because their joints are continually exposed to high sudden loads, but studies of these groups have not produced convincing evidence for this theory. They do get osteo-arthritis but then so do other groups who have not been exposed to this kind of exercise.

It is possible that, as is suspected in coronary heart disease, there are particularly susceptible individuals who are at risk and who cannot be identified until the disease becomes manifest and it is too late to do much about it. Their unknown presence obscures attempts to draw conclusions from population studies.

Exercise does appear to have two very important beneficial effects on the musculo-skeletal system. Strong muscles acting across a joint are necessary for the stability of a joint, and for ensuring that the joint does not receive abnormal loads during normal movements which may damage it. Secondly, the intermittent loading of a joint in rhythmic exercise stimulates the flow of lubricant into it thus maintaining friction at a minimum and protecting the joint from wear. If these two things are not maintained then the range of movement becomes severely limited and stiffness develops.

However, the amount of exercise required for maintenance is small. Moving a joint passively through its complete range of movement once a day will prevent it from becoming stiff. The maintenance of muscle strength requires rather more effort, but exercise requiring 80 per cent or more of the muscle's maximum force performed only once a day will be enough. This is why physiotherapists have worked out exercises (as distinct from exercise) which are designed to involve the use of all the muscle groups. These also appear in the better keep fit books. They are especially important in rehabilitation after immobilization or disuse of a limb and in maintaining good musculo-skeletal condition in the elderly. They ensure the redevelopment or maintenance of both muscle strength and joint flexibility. How much more exercise than this is needed to ensure an optimum amount of lubrication is not known.

It is possible therefore that exercise actually protects normal joints from osteo-arthritis; one study has shown a lower incidence in old age in competitive Finnish runners. They had begun training in adolescence and after many years of running had experienced far more rhythmic exercise than most people. Their incidence of arthritis was half that of normal controls of the same age. Running may protect where football does not because it produces less stress on the joints. The alternative explanation is that the runners are a select group of non-vulnerable individuals who therefore show a lower incidence of osteo-arthritis in old age.

It may be that exercise over and above the moderate amount which is adequate for optimum lubrication and maintenance of muscle strength is irrelevant. There is good evidence that osteo-arthritis is a late sequel to some specific joint damage or abnormality. Joints which have to accept abnormal or excessive loads during a lifetime either because of previous joint injury or abnormal growth are susceptible to osteo-arthritis. For example, in a study of 327 consecutive patients undergoing hip replacement all but 27 were found to have some abnormality attributable to previous damage.

Having once got osteo-arthritis, does exercise help or do harm? Gentle exercise will not do harm and it is necessary for the reasons already explained. It will not cure the condition but if muscle strength and joint flexibility and lubrication are not adequately maintained then the situation will get worse faster. Osteo-arthritis is a condition in which some pain and stiffness are inevitable. Exercise should be chosen which at least does not make the pain any worse. Swimming is particularly suitable because the cushioning effect of the water prevents sudden jarring stresses on the joints.

Rheumatoid arthritis is a very different disease. The cause is not entirely clear but it is a chronic disease affecting the whole body with acute damage to the tissues of many joints. The confusion between rheumatoid arthritis and osteo-arthritis may occasionally arise because the symptoms of painful joints are the same. During the acute phases of rheumatoid illness complete rest is necessary for recovery, and exercise would increase the severity of the joint damage. But when the acute inflammatory phase is in abeyance exercise can help for the normal reasons. It does not cure the condition but the gains in muscle strength and stamina can be achieved safely. After weeks of inactivity, exercise is an important factor in the struggle to maintain the quality of life in the face of a debilitating disease.

Osteoporosis is a condition which affects the skeleton. Bones consist of a protein framework which gains strength from calcium and other mineral salts laid down around it. Osteoporosis is said to have occurred when the protein framework begins to disappear and the calcium and salts with it. The bones are then more brittle and become inclined to break. This occurs to some extent with increasing age and to a greater degree in women than men.

It has been suggested that exercise might offset this age-based degeneration in bone, because of the way in which bone responds to extra loading by becoming denser. Normal bone depends for its maintenance on the pull of gravity and on the mechanical stimulation of muscles pulling on them. In abnormal conditions of inactivity, immobilization, and weightlessness, loss of bone substance occurs resulting in reduced bone density and loss of calcium. Much of the evidence for this comes from space research, but also lying in bed, for whatever reason, in a normal gravitational field with the legs horizontal leads to loss of bone substance which is prevented by allowing the patient to stand up or even sit for part of the day. It is not prevented by exercises in bed. Under normal conditions daily activity is sufficient to maintain bone density, and the bone loss which occurs with increasing age is not reduced by increased physical activity. The mean rate of mineral loss in women after the menopause is not constant with ageing. The greatest loss occurs in the youngest groups and since elderly women are usually less active, some factor other than decreased physical activity must account for the rates of mineral loss.

There is a case to be made for exercise in combating musculo-skeletal disorders, and the case against inactivity is even clearer. The extreme situation of complete immobilization, such as occurs in a plaster cast or when there is pain due to damage, results in loss of mobility, stiffness, and loss of strength in the muscles round the joint. This is particularly apparent in footballers who suffer cartilage damage to the knee joint. The strength and bulk of the thigh muscle disappears within days and places the joint at risk from further injury. It is therefore likely that inactivity of a less complete kind contributes to the development of joint stiffness and muscle weakness especially in the elderly. It may also be a cause of low back pain which affects 80 per cent of the world's population at some time. In 1979 a government department put the cost of back pain in the United Kingdom at £1 million a day, two-thirds of which is in lost industrial output and the rest in medical care.

For this reason, it has been suggested that physical activity can both prevent and cure back pain. However, since 92 per cent of these cases get better within two months, regardless of treatment, it is hard to be sure about the role of exercise. It should also be remembered that over-enthusiastic practising of weight-lifting or yoga exercises leads to excessive strains and can even produce back pain.

Exercises which relax the back muscles and strengthen the abdominal muscles are useful. Since all the limb muscles act against the support and opposition of the trunk muscles and since many of them are constantly at work as anti-gravity muscles they deserve attention. Almost any unfamiliar activity, even an un-usually long walk, leaves trunk muscles slightly stiff as well as the more obvious leg muscles. This shows that they too have been working harder than normal.

The strength of abdominal muscles is as important as the strength of the back muscles because they also help to maintain the trunk as a cylinder supporting the spine, for instance in lifting heavy objects. The thigh muscles take more weight when lifting correctly; the abdominal muscles are braced and the back is kept straight while the legs straighten from a bent position to pick up the load. This relieves the load on the spine and protects it from potential damage.

If you lift a weight of 27 kilograms (60 pounds) off the ground, bending the back and using the long levers of the trunk and arms, the back muscles have to balance that lifting force, but they must pull over the short distances between the vertebral bones so their mechanical advantage is poor and their strength must be great. (It is like trying to pull the door shut from the hinge end which is much harder than using the handle and the width of the door as the lever.) Meanwhile the vertebral disc may have to withstand a force of 500 kilograms (half a ton).

Low back pain is probably often muscular in origin and due to muscle tension or muscle spasm. Sciatica, lumbago, and fibrositis are due to pressure on trapped nerve roots which can happen if the resilient discs between the vertebrae wear out or slip out of place or if the muscles fail to hold the vertebrae in place. More working days are lost per year due to back pain than any other single disability. If exercise could prevent or cure it, it would save a great deal of money as well as misery.

11

EXERCISE AND DIABETES

Starving in the midst of plenty

This short chapter has been included because diabetes is an increasingly common disorder and because exercise is known to have a helpful effect on one kind of diabetes. It is even suspected that the increasing incidence of diabetes in Western societies is due partly to lack of exercise or to obesity, but there is no firm evidence.

Diabetes mellitus is a serious disorder of carbohydrate metabolism, often referred to colloquially as 'sugar' because it is characterized by loss of sugar in the urine. It is not to be confused with a much rarer condition called diabetes insipidus which is due to defective control of body water balance. Diabetes mellitus left untreated is a life-threatening condition; it cannot be cured but it can be effectively controlled by diet and exercise in mild cases or by the addition of insulin or one of its substitutes in more acute cases.

In the normal person, insulin is one of the hormones responsible for controlling the concentration of glucose in the blood by allowing glucose to enter the cells, especially muscle and adipose (fat) cells. In diabetes the passage of glucose into these cells is reduced because of lack of insulin or loss of sensitivity to it. As a consequence the concentration of glucose in the blood rises, especially after a meal, and overflows into the urine. Diabetics are sometimes therefore said to be starving in the midst of plenty.

This situation can arise for two reasons, in other words there are two forms of diabetes. If the disease developed in youth there is normally a lack of insulin production in the body. The pancreas where it is produced is unable to manufacture and release normal or appropriate amounts of insulin. In maturity-onset diabetes which occurs typically in middle-aged adults who are overweight there is no lack of insulin, in fact there may be more than usual circulating in the blood, but it is not effective in promoting the uptake of glucose by the cells. The cells are said to have become insulin resistant.

In both cases, both juvenile- and maturity-onset diabetes, the net results are the same. The blood glucose levels rise higher and stay high for longer after carbohydrate food, such as bread or sweets, has been eaten. At the same time this circulating glucose is not getting into the muscle cells where it is needed for energy release. The diabetic loses glucose in the urine and feels weak and tired because the muscles do not have adequate energy resources. Eventually such a person feels more and more unwell because the muscle cells produce toxic substances. These come from the inadequate breakdown of fats which goes on in order to release a little energy. ·

Exercise can help because it has an influence on the passage of glucose into muscle cells. Not only is this increased greatly during the exercise because glucose is being used up rapidly but there is also an increase for many hours afterwards. This is partly due to an increased effectiveness of insulin and the cells are said to have become more insulin sensitive. This effect of exercise is apparent both in normal people and in diabetics. The exercise has to be reasonably vigorous. A gentle stroll is no use, but brisk walking or jogging is effective. Conversely, complete bed-rest in normal people for several days reduces their rate of glucose uptake. They become more like diabetics.

Many maturity-onset diabetics can be effectively treated through diet and exercise and even juvenile diabetics who need insulin therapy can benefit from a carefully controlled exercise programme. They should not assume that vigorous exercise is impossible for them, although it does present some hazards if an adequate diet and insulin dosage are not properly balanced. There is a potential danger in severe exercise for those receiving injections of insulin for the following reason. The exercise will use up large quantities of glucose and at the same time there is no way of reducing the steady rate of flow of insulin into the blood from the injection depot under the skin. In fact the rate of flow increases during exercise because of the increased local blood flow through muscle and skin surrounding the injection site. The combination of exercise and insulin sometimes reduces the blood glucose concentration to such low levels that consciousness is lost because the brain is running short of its essential glucose supply. A sugar lump or a piece of chocolate restores blood glucose levels within ten to fifteen minutes and dramatic recovery follows.

Despite these difficulties most diabetics learn to cope with their impairment and adjust their diet and their insulin so that they can lead normal lives. They should not forget to include plenty of exercise in the equation and nor should the rest of us. It is better not to court diabetic symptoms at all than to have to live with them once the disease is established.

12

EXERCISE AND OBESITY

How fat is too fat?

Is it better to have the voluptuous curves of the women Rubens painted or to be as skinny as a twentieth-century photographer's model like Twiggy? Fashions change and reflect the economic climate of the time, but Ogden Nash's answer is as good as any and it holds for the men as well. He said,

> I like my women to be lithe and lissom
> But not so much that you cut yourself
> If you happen to embrace or kiss 'em.

If we favour being fat and happy, what is the come-uppance? Unfortunately there is a penalty; obesity may not be a disease in the normal sense but it is certainly not healthy to be fat.

Of course fat is useful. It is an energy store which is used continuously as well as glucose as an energy source. It is needed to spare the small glucose stores in prolonged strenuous exercise and in starvation, but quite small amounts are adequate for normal energy expenditure and even a bout of strenuous exercise is not going to use up more than a few hundred grams of fat. This will be replaced after the next meal since starvation is unlikely in Western countries apart from self-inflicted fasts. There is therefore no point in carrying about with us at least 20 kilograms (44 pounds) of fat which would enable us to survive weeks of semi-starvation. It is rather like burdening ourselves permanently with a rucksack full of spare clothes in case we fall in the river.

The burden of carrying about quantities of unnecessary fat stores can reduce the quality of life in various ways. First of all any physical activity in which the body weight is carried, such as walking or running, is more of an effort. Swimming and cycling will not be affected but walking upstairs makes extra weight especially noticeable. Being overweight can make physical activity a drag rather than a pleasure.

Physical appearance is not enhanced by rolls of fat and acceptable clothes which are also comfortable are hard to find. Women are probably more affected by these considerations but a flabby middle-aged man with a paunch and baggy trousers is not an attractive sight.

Worse than all this, obesity is associated with a higher incidence of certain diseases and a lower life expectancy. Maturity-onset diabetes mellitus, heart disease, and high blood pressure are chronic diseases which are more common among those who are overweight. Obesity increases the risk of death from these diseases and it is also a hazard if abdominal surgery is necessary. The fat gets in the surgeon's way and its presence can lead to various post-operative complications.

Everyone has some fat, but how much will lead to the possibility of these unpleasant consequences? The Metropolitan Life Insurance Company has kept records for many years of heights, weights, ages, and causes of death, and from this has compiled tables of desirable weights for any specified height and build. Desirable weights are those associated with the lowest death rates. If you are more than 20 per cent over that desirable weight then your risk of death is increased.

Having admitted that they are overweight and that something must be done about it people sometimes 'go on a diet', but this is not the simple solution that it seems. The daily calorie intake can be reduced by having smaller helpings or by eating lettuce instead of suet pudding and oranges instead of cream cakes. This works if the diet is sensibly balanced containing enough protein and vitamins, if the reduction in calories is not too drastic, and if there is sufficient strength of mind to turn away from the forbidden sweet or fatty things. Losing weight on a low-calorie diet is a miserable business and sufficient will-power to resist temptation is often lacking. Then even if the diet is faithfully followed and the requisite amount of weight lost there is normally a return to previous eating habits and in a few weeks it is back again. Unless there is a permanent change in eating habits, 'diets' will never be an effective long-term method of weight control.

An alternative solution which might be less unpleasant and so more successful is to take more physical exercise, to increase the expenditure of calories instead of decreasing the intake. Exercise has been neglected as a means of controlling weight because its effects are small and therefore slow. Nevertheless it deserves to be

Table 1. Desirable weight for height

Males		Females	
Height cm	Weight range kg	Height cm	Weight range kg
145	51.9 – 54.4	140	44.9 – 47.1
146	52.4 – 55.0	141	45.4 – 47.6
147	52.9 – 55.5	142	45.9 – 48.1
148	53.5 – 56.1	143	46.4 – 48.7
149	54.0 – 56.7	144	47.0 – 49.3
150	54.5 – 57.2	145	47.5 – 49.8
151	55.0 – 57.7	146	48.0 – 50.3
152	55.6 – 58.3	147	48.6 – 51.0
153	56.1 – 58.9	148	49.2 – 51.6
154	56.6 – 59.4	149	49.8 – 52.2
155	57.2 – 60.0	150	50.4 – 52.9
156	57.9 – 60.7	151	51.0 – 53.5
157	58.6 – 61.5	152	51.5 – 54.0
158	59.3 – 62.2	153	52.0 – 54.5
159	59.9 – 62.8	154	52.5 – 55.1
160	60.5 – 63.5	155	53.1 – 55.7
161	61.1 – 64.1	156	53.7 – 56.3
162	61.7 – 64.7	157	54.3 – 57.0
163	62.3 – 65.4	158	54.9 – 57.6
164	62.9 – 66.0	159	55.5 – 58.2
165	63.5 – 66.6	160	56.3 – 59.0
166	64.0 – 67.1	161	56.9 – 59.7
167	64.6 – 67.8	162	57.6 – 60.4
168	65.2 – 68.4	163	58.3 – 61.2
169	65.9 – 69.1	164	58.9 – 61.8
170	66.6 – 69.9	165	59.5 – 62.4
171	67.3 – 70.6	166	60.1 – 63.1
172	68.0 – 71.3	167	60.7 – 63.7
173	68.7 – 72.1	168	61.4 – 64.4
174	69.4 – 72.8	169	62.1 – 65.1
175	70.1 – 73.6		
176	70.8 – 74.3		
177	71.6 – 75.1		
178	72.4 – 76.0		
179	73.3 – 76.9		
180	74.2 – 77.9		
181	75.0 – 78.7		
182	75.8 – 79.5		
183	76.5 – 80.3		
184	77.3 – 81.1		
185	78.1 – 81.9		
186	78.9 – 82.8		

Notes: 1. Height in inches multiplied by 2.5 gives height in centimetres.
      2. Weight in pounds divided by 2.2 gives weight in kilograms.
Source: *The Assessment of the Nutritional Status of the Community*, D. B. Jelliffe, W.H.O., 1966. (Adapted by permission from Society of Actuaries (1959) – modified for average frame size and nude measurements.)

reconsidered, not as a substitute for a sensible diet but in addition. If it is part of a two-pronged 'fight against the flab' the reduction in calorie intake can be less severe and long-term defeat of the enemy is much more likely.

The reasons why people become fat are not well understood. It is often assumed that those who are fat have become so through gluttony. This is not necessarily so and no one has been able to find any evidence for it. It is just as likely that they have become fat by eating the same amount as other people but doing less. Intake must equal expenditure, the rules which apply to monetary budgets also apply to calories. It is sometimes said that thin people act first and think afterwards and that fat people think first and act afterwards thus avoiding a good deal of unnecessary activity. Maybe it is the fidgeting and 'unnecessary' activity which keeps the thin people thin.

There is some evidence to support this in that fat children are found to be less active than their thin contemporaries and over-weight adults are also less active than their lean counterparts.

These differences only appear if activity levels are measured objectively using cine film or pedometers. Questionnaires have not shown up clear-cut differences. They are notoriously unreliable and do not reveal differences because either the lean individuals think they do less than they really do or the fat individuals think they do more.

The implications of this difference in activity levels are not straightforward. The total energy expended by an obese person will be greater than by a thin person for any given activity because of the extra weight the obese person carries around. Thus the less active obese individuals may well expend just as much energy as the more active lean. This tallies with the evidence that there is no significant difference in the amounts of food that fat and thin people eat. However, if the obese want to lose weight then either they must eat less or they must do more, or better still, both.

Many people reject exercise as a way of losing weight because they think it increases appetite. This is not true; it can sometimes reduce it directly because one does not feel hungry immediately after exercise or indirectly because an exercise programme makes one feel more health conscious in other ways. The prodigious meals which some of us eat on holiday after a day on the beach owe more to the general holiday atmosphere, the social scene, and having time to enjoy a leisurely meal than to an increase in activity.

An extra half-an-hour's walk per day will only use up a few grams of fat but if this becomes a routine then, after a year, 6 kilograms (14 pounds) of fat may have gone. Moreover, the extra exercise improves exercise tolerance, so the extra walk becomes more of a pleasure and less of a burden. It is to be hoped that this will lead to more or faster walking which will compensate for the reduction in energy expenditure as body weight drops. If this seems slow, consider how much pleasanter it is than life without any chocolates, pastry, or chips. Inclusion of exercise does leave some scope for occasional indulgence.

Sometimes the weight loss with exercise is greater than would be predicted from the energy cost of the activity and it seems possible that exercise may have a general stimulating effect on the body which persists throughout the day, raising the resting rate of energy expenditure and burning up even more calories. This is an exciting possibility. If exercise increases metabolic rate and makes us less efficient then it will be much easier to control weight through modest dieting.

No attempt at severe dieting with or without exercise should be made without consultation with a doctor. Total starvation leads to disastrous loss of protein as well as fat. Protein starvation is generally harmful to the heart and liver.

The kinds of exercise most likely to help with weight control are the rhythmic endurance ones which use large muscles and burn up the most calories. These include walking, running, rambling, hill-climbing, swimming, cycling, and many sports and ball games. Weight-lifting or weight-training will not be of much use for losing weight.

If obesity is associated with increased risk of disease, does a reduction in weight lead to a reduction in risk? It is certainly true that when an obese person loses weight, blood pressure and blood levels of cholesterol come down, and this is likely to reduce the long-term risk of death or disability from stroke and heart disease. Exercise also improves the way in which glucose is handled as explained in the last chapter and so the risk is reduced of developing the form of diabetes which occurs in later life.

It is undoubtedly true that it is healthier to be skinny. If weight can be lost with exercise, then reducing diets need not be so extreme. Life will be much pleasanter with a few more calories for lunch and a well-trained muscle system to take you out afterwards.

13

IN CONCLUSION

These chapters have been written in an endeavour to answer as honestly as possible the many questions which are constantly asked about exercise and its value. Many of the answers are old fashioned and the reasons for them sometimes complicated. In presenting the answers we have tried to avoid both specialist obscurantism and popular proselytizing.

We were reluctant to foist upon our readers a set of doctrinaire opinions based upon interesting hypotheses rather than soundly established fact. Jogging is often greeted cynically as just another health fad, here today and gone tomorrow like monkey gland and Queen Bee jelly. So we have indicated which are the facts for which there is good evidence and which are our own informed guesses in areas where evidence is circumstantial or totally lacking.

Some of the answers are still missing. Academics should not be allowed to use this as an excuse to retreat into their ivory towers and to refuse the attempt to provide at least the best available answers.

Having consulted the experts in many fields and read the available literature, we have come off the fence firmly in favour of exercise. We are quite certain about this provided that we add the warning that the exercise be sensibly pursued.

The argument that man is endowed with muscles and therefore should use them sounds convincing, but it does not prove that exercise is necessary. However, there is plenty of other evidence which has been presented in these chapters for the very real benefits which exercise brings. In the end each man or woman must convince himself or herself. Therefore we cannot advocate too strongly that, having given the case for exercise a hearing, you give the exercise a try.

This will involve changing personal priorities, but it may involve a financial commitment. However, the cost of a good pair of running shoes is small compared to the amounts spent on alcohol, tobacco, and entertainment.

Activity levels tend to drift imperceptibly downwards in affluent Western society and if the deterioration is noticed at all it is usually considered to be inevitable. It is not until an abrupt change, hopefully in the direction of increased activity and better physical condition, occurs that we realize how far from the optimum we have let ourselves get.

Despite these remarks, we would also emphasize that if you decide to become more active, there are three cardinal rules. Do it reasonably gradually; do it in a way that fits into your regular routine; and do something which you will enjoy, once you are used to it, if not straight away.

The public image of exercise is improving, but it is sad that in many quarters it is still seen as something penal, a punishment to be meted out to miscreant youth. The courts send young offenders to detention centres where they are drilled in strenuous physical exercises instead of being free to watch the local football match. We have not come far yet from the treadmills of Victorian prisons. It is no wonder that the virtuous middle-aged regard exercise at the best as undignified, and at the worst as degrading.

Let us hope that the microchip will usher in an age when paradoxically the extra leisure will enable us to rediscover our muscles and regain a youthful zest for living. Youth is hardly ever lost. Don't relegate it to the back of the cupboard for ever.

Exercise can
Enhance normal health
Prevent disease
Ameliorate the effects of disease

FURTHER READING

Popular books

Carruthers, M. and Murray, A. *F/40 Fitness on 40 Minutes a Week* (Futura Publications, 1976)

Cooper, K. H. *The New Aerobics* (Bantam Books, 1970)

Mann, J. *Walk! A Handbook* (Paddington Press, 1979)

Michener, L. and Donaldson, G. *The Exercise Book* (Penguin, 1978)

Mossfeldt, F. and Miller, M. S. *In-the-Chair Exercise Book* (Bantam Books, 1979)

Oram, C. *Everywoman* (World's Work, 1978)

Oram, C. *Going Well Over Sixty* (World's Work, 1979)

Pontefract, R. (ed.) *Feel Fit – Come Alive* (Oxford University Press, 1979)

Prowse, D. *Fitness is Fun* (W. H. Allen, 1979)

Royal Canadian Air Force *Physical Fitness* (Penguin, 1970)

Tulloh, B. *The Complete Jogger* (Pan Books, 1979)

Specialist books

Astrand, P. O. and Rodahl, K. *Textbook of Work Physiology* (McGraw-Hill, 1977)

Getchell, B. *Physical Fitness. A Way of Life* (Wiley, 1976)

Morehouse, L. E. and Miller, A. T. *Physiology of Exercise* (Mosby, 1976)

Shephard, R. J. *Frontiers of Fitness* (Thomas, 1971)

Shephard, R. J. *Human Physiological work Capacity* (Cambridge University Press, 1978)

Shephard, R. J. *Physical Activity and Aging* (Croom Helm, 1978)

Recent publications

The Good Health Guide, The Open University in association with the Health Education Council and the Scottish Health Education Unit (Harper & Row, 1980)

INDEX

Numbers in italic refer to the main discussion of a topic